A Calculus of Curing

Copyright: Tracy D Kolenchuk, 2018-2019
Editor: Catherine Owen
All Rights Reserved

ISBN-13: 978-1986878425

ISBN-10: 1986878422

This book is a black and white edition of the book:
CURE
and
An expansion of the concepts in the paper:
A Theory of Cure
and the book
The Elements of Cure

Food for thought.

> **US/FDA Nonsense Warning**
>
> *This book is not intended to "diagnose, treat, cure or prevent any disease... because only a drug can legally make such a claim" (US/FDA Label Claims for Conventional Foods and Dietary Supplements).*

Seriously? No. Legally? Yes. Only a drug can claim to cure.

This book begins
a journey to understanding cure,
to cure illnesses
with health,
because only health can cure.

This book is not about medicine,
nor about alternative medicine.

It's a healthicine book.

A book about cures and the concept of curing.

Dedication:

To my mom, Irene Kolenchuk, who has been incorrectly diagnosed and treated for many medical conditions and diseases for over 60 years still waits for an answer.

The Healthicine Creed

Health is whole. Health is wide and deep.
Health is slow and steady.
Health is honest and true.
Health enables freedoms. Freedoms enable health.
Health encompasses all life processes, from genetics to Gaia.

Health is a verb. *To health* is to make healthier.
Health is a noun: A healthiness is a measurable instance of health.
An unhealthiness is a potential for improvement in health.

An illness is a hole in the health of body, mind, spirit or community.
An illness consists of a present cause, and it's negative consequences.
Every illness is a judgment.
Causal illnesses have present active process causes.
Injury illnesses are holes in body, mind, spirit or community.
Attribute illnesses are caused by attributes of diet, body, mind, spirits or community.
Chronic illnesses have chronic causes.
Symptomicines can create and facilitate chronic illnesses.

Every illness can be cured.
Causal cures stop the progression of a causal illness.
Healing cures repair damage and defend against illness.
Transformations cure attribute illnesses, often requiring healing.

Health is the best preventative.

Everyone has a right to life, liberty, and the pursuit of healthiness.

Preface

This is a book about the word cure, the many concepts of cure. No current practice of medicine has a clear, general definition of cure.

Today's official medical systems go by many names: conventional medicine, modern medicine, allopathic medicine, mainstream medicine, orthodox medicine, and more. In this text, I use the term conventional medicine. Conventional medicine is a practice, not a science, and I will often use the term medical practice – there being no generally accepted theories nor sciences of medicine.

Much of conventional medicine is well, conventional. It functions as a powerful bureaucracy, as described by Eric Fromm in To Have or To Be, *"The bureaucratic method can be defined as one that a) administers human beings as if they were things and b) administers things in a quantitative rather than qualitative terms ... governed by statistical data.... Base their decisions on fixed rules arrived from statistical data, rather than on response to the living beings who stand before them... at the risk of hurting the 5 or 10 percent of those who do not fit into that pattern. Bureaucrats fear responsibility and seek refuge behind their rules; their security and pride lie in their loyalty to the rules, not in their loyalty to the laws of the human heart."*

Many have observed that conventional medicine functions best in the emergency department. Emergency medicine, like wartime medicine, has little use for convention. In emergencies, every patient is a unique case, not a statistic. Every case is an anecdote, not a clinical study. There are no diseases to diagnose. The doctor must act based on the patient and their condition and is seldom able to rely on statistical data about treatments recommended in clinical studies. Conventional medicine shines when the bureaucratic factor is lowest. On the other hand, conventional medicine, bureaucratic medicine, is a complete failure with regards to chronic illnesses. Conventional medicine defines chronic diseases without logic: *"A chronic disease... is a disease lasting three months or longer."* (National Mental Health Council) and *"Chronic diseases are defined broadly as conditions that last 1 year or more and require ongoing medical attention or limit activities of daily living or both."* (National Center for Chronic Disease Prevention and Health Promotion). All chronic diseases are spoken of and treated as incurable. The rise in incurable chronic disease is directly linked to the growth of bureaucracy in medicine.

Conventional medicine has no concept of cured for most medical conditions. Most diseases cannot be cured, *"by lack of definition."* Evidence Based Medicine, one of the latest trends, is an extremely bureaucratic medicine, based entirely on statistical results. Cure is not defined in Evidence Based Medicine either.

The inability or unwillingness to define cure has resulted in an ongoing nonsense competition between so-called *conventional medical treatments and techniques* and so-called *alternative medical treatments and techniques* debating *which DOES NOT CURE better.* We should not judge by the name, nor the history, nor philosophy of a treatment, but by results. Is the illness cured?

To understand cure, we might consult the experts, but there are none. Who are the medical experts who can explain cure, cures, curing, and cured? What are the medical journals devoted to studying the theory and practices of curing? There are none. Medical journals focus on prevention and treatments for diseases assumed to be incurable. If we can cure a disease, there is little need for a journal. What organization represents the experts on curing any curable disease? There are none.

Who studies cures? The question is not an Abbott and Costello skit. WHO, the World Health Organization makes no attempt to study cures. We have no idea who's on first, nor what's on second... *"I don't know"* is certainly on third when it comes to cures.

When we define the concept of cured for every illness and develop and study a calculus of curing, we can judge every medical practice on a level field of cures.

As we work to define cure, cures, curing, and cured, we need to create new words and phrases. Words like illness, disease, and cure have a long and complex history. They are too vague to articulate any understanding of curing or to facilitate scientific scrutiny.

Who am I?

Why me, you might ask, who am I to write about cure? I am neither a doctor nor a scientist. I can only respond: Who else will do it? Who else has ever tried? No one.

This book began with a problem. One afternoon, in July of 2016, I was browsing the shelves of a used bookstore near the University, looking for clues to the concepts of cure. I had been working to revise the book Introduction to Healthicine, published several years ago, and I was stuck. I got stuck on the word cure. I could not find a useful definition anywhere.

I spotted the Webster's New World Medical Dictionary, 3rd edition. I picked it off the shelf and opened it to the letter C. I scanned, *"cultural revolution, culture, curettage."* What? I turned the page, looking for cure. *Cure* was not in the dictionary. I turned to the letter i, looking for incurable. Not there either. I was stunned. A prestigious medical dictionary did not contain entries for cure, cures, cured, curing, nor incurable. A more recent edition contains a definition of cure, but it's a historical, not a medical one.

The next day, I visited a local Chapters bookstore, in search of more medical dictionaries. Many did not contain entries for the word cure. The few that did contained simplistic entries, like those in non-medical dictionaries. I found that cure does not appear in Barron's Dictionary of Medical Terms, Sixth Edition, 2013, although incurable is defined as *"being such that a cure is impossible within the realm of known medical practice."* Since then, I have written and continue to write many posts about cure and developing my ideas through blogging. Some of those posts have been updated as I write and edit this book.

I had been researching the word cure for a few years already, and had checked a few dictionary definitions, and blogged about them. I'd checked more than a few major medical reference texts, to see what they said about cure. Almost nothing. I'd visited the University Library archives and checked the Merck Manual of Diagnosis and Therapy as far back as the 1950s. I had read the entire first edition of Merck and checked every instance of the word cure in the 11th Edition of Merck. I hadn't learned much, except that the word cure is poorly defined if at all. No medical reference provides a useful, scientific definition of cure.

I was already aware that cure is not defined and not in the index of most, if not all, major medical references, including The Merck Manual of Diagnosis and Therapy, Harrison's Guide to Internal Medicine, Lange's Current Medical Diagnosis and Treatment, and Ferri's Clinical Advisor.. The DSM-5, the Diagnostic and Statistical Manual of Mental Disorders does not contain the word cure in the index nor anywhere in the text except an introductory hope *"eventual cures for these conditions."* We might conclude that all conditions listed in the DSM-5 are incurable by the absence of a definition of cured.

I gradually learned that the word cure is not just avoided but forbidden in many medical practices. Conventional medicine has serious problems with the word cure. There is no current general medical theory. Therefore; there is no current medical theory of cure. There are cures, of course, and reference books like the Merck Manual of Diagnosis and Therapy occasionally use the word cure. However, use of the word cure, in all medical references, is weak and inconsistent. Almost half of the references to cure in Merck are *incurable* and variations of *cannot be cured.* Incurable is also not defined. Without a definition, conventional medicine cannot prove most diseases cured or not cured.

It took a long time for me to realize that the word *cured*, which is not in medical dictionaries either, has many distinct meanings. We need definitions of cured that fit each disease, if we are to cure any case and know that it has been cured.

Is this a recent occurrence? No. The Lexicon Medicum, Seventh Edition, also known as Hooper's Medical Dictionary, 1838 offers "*CURATIO. Cura. The treatment of a disease or injury. It is not synonymous with our word cure; since it applies to a treatment whether successful or otherwise; thus, curare vulnis does not mean to cure a wound, but to dress a wound."* But does not provide a definition for cure. The London Medical Dictionary, published in 1819, uses the word cure several times but does not provide a definition. Cure, it appears, was not defined in 1818, and 200 years later, it is still not defined. In the original version of Merck´s 1899 Manual of the Materia Médica several cures are recommended. Most are nonsense with a single exception: iridectomy. In the 1950s cure hardly appeared in Merck, was not defined, and not used consistently.

According to the US/FDA labelling guidelines for Structure/Function claims, no one can claim a cure for any nutritional product, unless they also *"say how widespread such a disease is in the United States… because only a drug can legally make such a claim"* (to diagnose, treat, cure or prevent any disease). Conventional medicine has no definitions of cures. Bureaucrats pass laws against them. The US/FDA claim that only medicines can cure has led to an epidemic of medical chauvinism, strongly supported by drug manufacturers producing and marketing products that make no attempt to cure.

> *Equally problematic to medical chauvinism is "scientism," which is the common assumption that science is the only way to acquire knowledge about reality.*
> *- Dana Ullman*

Incurable Diseases
Are any diseases incurable? There have been many nonsensical suggestions with no scientific foundation. Years ago, Wikipedia had a

page with an extensive list of incurable diseases. In 2010, this page was removed. Why? According to Wiki editors, *"this is a list with no clear-cut criteria for inclusion,"* and *"the lack of any sourcing to indicate that the majority of these are indeed considered incurable."* One editor commented *"Absolutely pointless grab-bag of medical conditions. No attempt at referencing. Unlikely to ever become useful."* As I write this section in 2017, Wikipedia has a new list of incurable diseases, created in 2016. It's still nonsense, even as it is frequently updated. The nonsense begins in the first two sentences, which contradict each other: *"This list is incomplete; you can help by expanding it."* followed by: *"This is a comprehensive list of incurable diseases. It includes both physical and mental diseases."* Note: this second sentence has been removed since then. Wikipedia's authors are building a new list of incurable diseases without defining incurable. Most diseases are considered incurable at present. Diseases are not defined to facilitate a definition of cured and cured is not defined medically. Incurable says more about the system than about any disease.

The concept of disease is a powerful tool in medicine. Assigning a name, by diagnosis, gives the doctor, and the patient, something to reference, study, and research. We study diseases in different cases, across the timespan of the disease, decades, even centuries. When a doctor diagnoses a case of disease, they can prepare a prognosis and a treatment plan, based on a documented history.

The concept of disease also creates many problems. We use the word disease to refer to a single case of a disease and to the general concept of a group of diseases. A single case of a disease might be cured, but a disease, a general class of illnesses, cannot be cured.

Every illness is a single case, whether it is diagnosed as a disease or not makes little difference. Only an illness can be cured. Every cure is an individual, unique story, an anecdote.

An Apology to Doctors

I am not a doctor. My life has been saved by doctors on more than one occasion. This book is not written to diminish in any way the intelligence, hard work, and valuable services provided by doctors.

This book aims to change, to enhance, encourage, and to prod a medical system that refuses to acknowledge cures, much less to study cure scientifically.

This book is about cure, not about medicine, not about the practices of medicine. Cures come from health. This is a healthicine book, a book about health.

I write in the hope that someday, studies of health, and studies of cures, will become valuable parts of our practices of medicine. When that happens, many medical treatments will disappear, along with them many negative side effects, adverse consequences, and iatrogenic illnesses.

To your health, tracy

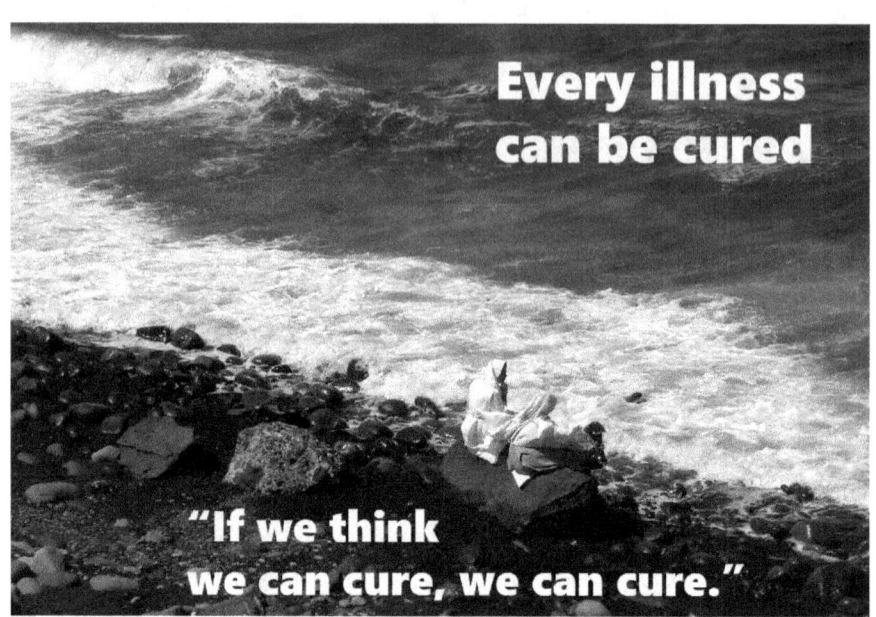

that's the spirit

The Meaning of Cure 1

Do Medicines Cure? 15

Illness, Disease, Sickness 23

Elements of Illness 41

Elements of Cause 45

Composite Illnesses 72

Signs and Symptoms 93

Elements of Cure 99

Health is Whole 109

Illness: A Hole in Healthiness 115

Judgements and Closure 121

Cures 133

Curing Causal Illness 181

Curing Injury Illness 185

Curing Attribute Illness 195

Curing Chronic Illness 213

Circles of Illness, Causes, and Cures 229

Cured 235

To Have an Illness, or To Be Ill 243

Summary and Conclusions 245

Epilogue: Books That Cure 255

Appendix: Definitions 273

The Meaning of Cure

There are no such things as incurables; there are only things for which man has not found a cure.
— *Bernard M Baruch*

Two doctors meet in the hospital cafeteria. Jan is an old hand, crusty and a bit intolerant of silliness. Jamie is a new intern, just out of school. They've paired up together for work, and lunches. As they sit down, Jamie feels the glow of excitement of becoming a doctor.

"I can hardly wait to start curing people," Jamie gushes.

"Cure? What do you mean by cure?" Jan asks sternly.

"You know, to help them get rid of their diseases. To free people from disease." Jamie is speaking rapidly, enthusiastically.

"Maybe you should check a dictionary," Jan replies curtly.

"What?"

"Well, if you check your dictionary, you might be surprised at the meaning of cure. Take note of disease as well. Illness is what the patient has. Disease is a classification system used for diagnosis and statistics. Not every illness can be diagnosed as a disease. Not every diagnosis is correct. And cure? That's a real challenge."

Jamie types into the phone for a moment and reads, triumphantly: *"Cure: **'the act of making someone healthy again after an illness'** according to Webster."*

"Curing happens after the illness is gone?" Jan challenges, *"I thought that was healing? Doesn't curing happen when the patient is sick?*

Are you sure that's what Webster says?"

"Hmm," Jamie is flustered, *"Google shows the definition from the Learner's Dictionary first,"* she fumbles a bit, scrolling down.

CURE

Webster's online dictionary for English learners:

"the act of making someone healthy again after an illness"

| no illness | illness | after illness |

cure

© Healthicine

"So, first we give learners the wrong definition for cure, then correct it when they learn better English?" Jan smiles sarcastically. *"By the way, we don't make patients healthy, we treat them for serious medical conditions, and send them home, to heal. Health is not a medical issue."*

"Here," replies Jamie, attempting to move the conversation in a positive direction, *"it says... well, it's complicated."*

Jan provides a bit of support, *"There are lots of different meanings for the word cure, in different situations. But you said you want to get busy 'curing people.' Is there a definition like that?"*

*"It says **'to stop (a disease) by using drugs or other medical treatments**,' that's what I meant."* Jan smiles, then adds, shaking her head, *"then it says, again, **'the act of making someone healthy again after an illness.'"***

CURE

Webster's Dictionary

"to make (someone) healthy again after an illness"
"to stop (a disease) by using drugs or other medical treatments"

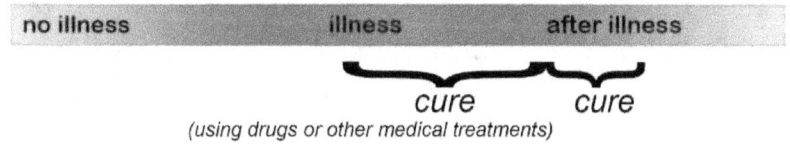

© Healthicine

"Curing someone is stopping their disease. That makes sense, although they've switched from illness to disease. Do we cure the illness, or the disease, or the patient? What if something stops the disease, but doesn't make them healthy, is it a cure?" Jan queries.

"You're just getting technical now, being pedantic." Jamie grins

"We could look up pedantic too, but let's stick to cure. The first definition is simply nonsense- healing after an illness doesn't cure an illness. Healing is part of growth, always active, before, during and after an illness. Healing progresses irrespective of the illness or disease, also irrespective of the cause, because healing repairs injuries, not diseases. The other definition is OK, except for the medicine restriction."

"Restriction?" Jamie seems puzzled.

*"It is, of course, possible to cure an illness, without a **'drug or medical treatment,'"*** Jan taps a knife on the tray for emphasis. *"That definition is a clear case of medical chauvinism."*

"Like, give me an example!" Jamie challenges.

"How do you cure simple dehydration? " Jan asks, smiling.

"Hmm...technically, dehydration is cured with water - I guess it's not a medicine, nor a medical treatment, except, when you are dehydrated, then it's a medical treatment!" Jamie responds.

"Well, that's nonsense. What if you are only partly dehydrated - is it a medicine? What if you self-diagnose and self-treat, is it a medicine? Is it a medicine if a doctor prescribes it, or if a medical person recommends it, but otherwise not? Is a bottle of water a medicine if the label says, **'can be used to prevent, treat, or cure dehydration,'** but not if it says **'pure, healthy, spring water'**? Lots of illnesses are cured without medicines. Many are cured by the presence of something, others by an absence, or by removing the cause. Obesity, arsenic poisoning, and shin splints are not cured by something. They can only be cured by not something. Even some infections can only be cured by surgically removing the infecting bacteria."

Jan continues, "*Of course dehydration is not usually a disease - it's usually a symptom of another problem. Giving water as a medicine doesn't address the cause. Dehydration caused by lack of water is rare because our bodies tell us when we need to drink water. Simple dehydration is normally cured by health before diagnosis.*"

"*An illness can be cured by health?*" Jamie looks surprised.

"*By actions that make you healthier. Lots of things are essential to health. If you don't get them, or don't get enough, you get sick - if you get too much, you get sick. Health is about balance, and the ability to maintain and make use of the balances of life.*" Jan replies, adding, "*Maybe we need a better dictionary.*"

"*I'll check Oxford,*" Jamie proposes, thumbing the phone again, "The Oxford Dictionary for English Learners: **'to make a person or an animal healthy again after an illness**,' duh - almost exactly the same as Webster's. Why do dictionaries think curing happens after the illness?"

"Dictionaries don't create language - they attempt to document how language is used. Writing a learner's dictionary is more difficult. They need to simplify, which can easily lead to simple errors. What does the full definition say?" Jan asks.

"I'm reading it, but I'm not liking it," Jamie replies, "It says **'relieve (a person or animal) of the symptoms of a disease or condition.'** But, we don't cure symptoms, do we?"

"There's often confusion between the symptoms of disease and actual illness." Jan pauses, thoughtfully.

Jamie interrupts, "Then it says **'Eliminate (a disease or condition) with medical treatment.'** Oxford also misses cures without medicines. Is there no logical, scientific, medical definition of cure?"

"Well, lunch is almost over - why don't you check some medical books. Maybe you'll find a better definition. Let's talk more about this tomorrow." Jan picks up the empty dishes and places them on a tray.

But before they leave the cafeteria, Jan has to ask, "What do you think cure means now?"

"I think cure means to stop the illness," Jamie replies.

"That's a good start," Jan replies, "Let's see what tomorrow brings."

The next day, Jan and Jamie are finishing up the morning rounds and heading to the hospital cafeteria. Jan re-opens yesterday's conversation.

"Well, did you learn anything about cure in your research last night?"

Jamie is frustrated, *"I learned that medical dictionaries don't take the word cure seriously."*

"Really? For example?" Jan picks up a tray and orders a Reuben.

"Well, first I went to Webster's New World Medical Dictionary, third edition. I had it in my office, a gift from a friend," Jamie pauses as she orders a sandwich.

"and..."

"Cure is not in the dictionary. Not cure, cured, cures, curing, nor curable. The definitions leap from culture to curettage. Not only that, incurable isn't defined either," Jamie sighs.

"That's just silly," Jan smirks sarcastically. *"Or maybe, you're on to something?"*

"It's ridiculous," Jamie agrees. *"At first, I thought maybe it was because Webster's Medical Dictionary, Third Edition, was newly prepared from the internet – a simple mistake..."*

"But?"

"Well, then I started checking more medical dictionaries. Lots of them, from The Oxford Concise Medical Dictionary to Medical Terminology for Dummies, do not contain the cure. Barron's Dictionary of Medical Terms does not define cure even though it defines incurable as **'being such that a CURE is impossible within the realm of known medical practice.'"**

"Hilarious," Jan snorts, *"do any medical dictionaries define cure?"*

"Yes, I found a few. Stedman's gives several definitions. The first one is **'to heal, to make well.'** But healing, as we've already discussed, happens before, during, and after the illness - independent of disease. And **'to make well'** is simplistic, less defined than cure."

CURE

Stedman's Medical Dictionary

"1. To heal, to make well."
"2. A restoration to health."
"3. A special method or course of treatment."

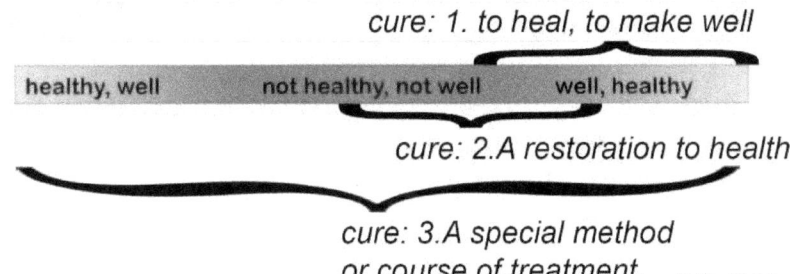

"I can see that. To make well, might range from an apology, intending to make the patient feel better, to a painkiller that helps them feel less pain, to an actual cure." Jan observes. "But doesn't 'well' mean without illness?"

Jamie responds, "That's OK in simple cases, but what if someone has more than one illness. Like, an older adult who suffers from obesity, hypertension, arthritis, and diabetes. If well is without illness, then, the Stedman's definition implies you can't cure one illness, because the patient is still not yet well."

"Now you're sounding technical and pedantic," Jan comments dryly.

"If we are to define cure, we need a definition that handles simple challenges," Jamie goes on, "the second definition is **'a restoration of health'** Does health disappear when someone gets sick?"

"Health is always present, as long as we are alive. Maybe they mean 'some health is lost' when we get sick, and we recover it when we get better." Jan offers.

"But, if restoration of health comes from healing, they're still mixing and confusing healing and curing" Jamie objects, but then continues, "their third definition is **'a special method or course of treatment'** It seems OK at first, but special is not defined. Most treatments are designed to address signs and symptoms. Most medical treatments do not cure. In fact, a 'course of treatment,' might be given to someone who is not sick, not in need of a cure. If someone gets a spa treatment, or a hair treatment, it doesn't mean they are sick, searching for a cure."

"So, Stedman's Medical Dictionary defines cures used when you are not sick, when you are sick, and after your sickness is gone. Is that so bad?"

"It's worse. They don't even use the word disease or illness. Can you cure someone who doesn't have an illness?" Jamie shows Jan her phone, enlarging the text, "how can we cure people, how can we search for cures if cure is not properly defined? How can we know if someone is cured, if cured is not in the medical dictionary? Can there be a science of medicine, if we don't have a scientific definition for cure?"

Jan responds quietly, "Did you check anywhere else?"

"Mosbey's Medical Dictionary is different but no better. They first define cure as **'restoration to health of a person afflicted with a disease or disorder'**."

"At least it mentions disease," Jan comments, "but not illness," he adds.

"Yes, but it's the same **'restoration to health**,' which implies that once you have a disease or a disorder, you are no longer healthy. Health doesn't disappear because you have an illness. If you lose your health – aren't you are dead?"

"Well, many diseases are the result of a decrease in health, and a *restoration of health is the only real cure. Scurvy is caused by an unhealthy diet and cured by a healthy diet."*

"Yes," Jamie agrees. *"It almost seems they recognized that restoring health can cure a disease - but I don't think they meant it that way."* She elaborates, *"It doesn't actually speak about stopping the illness. How can it be a cure if the illness isn't stopped?"*

Jan interrupts, *"Careful there. An illness is not a physical thing. It's not moving. Illness is an invisible concept. Illness exists when a cause results in signs and symptoms of disease. We cure by addressing the cause or the connection – and the illness, the invisible concept, disappears."*

"I haven't seen a single definition of cure that mentions cause. It's as if all diseases are caused by evil monsters. And what is a disorder?" Jamie queries, *"An amputated leg is a disorder - but we don't cure it. Mosbey's definition, like all the others, is useless as a medical or scientific tool."*

"Yes, we don't cure disabilities, only illnesses. Do they give another definition?" asks Jan.

CURE
Mosbey's Medical, Nursing, and Allied Health Dictionary

"1. Restoration to health of a person afflicted with a disease or other disorder."

"2. The favorable outcome of the treatment of a disease or other disorder."

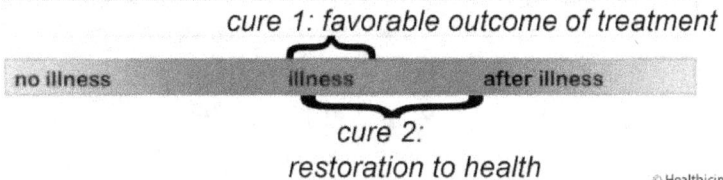

"'The favorable outcome of a treatment of a disease or disorder.' It's simplistic nonsense. A person has arthritis, and they take a medicine which makes them feels better, it's a favorable outcome. So, the medicine cured them, according to Mosbey's. But they still have arthritis, and it's probably getting worse." Jamie is visibly frustrated, stops talking and looks at Jan, hoping for an answer.

"Hmm..." Jan thinks aloud, *"So, Stedman's doesn't require an illness to define a cure, and Mosbey's does not require stopping the illness to qualify as a cure. It reminds me of the old joke, 'the operation was a success, but the patient died anyway.'"* Jan grins, *"if the cure is successful, and the patient is still sick? Is it a cure?"*

"It's worse. A favorable outcome as defined by the doctor? or by the patient? What if the patient's goals and the doctor's goals are different?" Jamie asks, rhetorically adding, *"A favorable outcome is not always a cure, even though a cure is almost always a favorable outcome."*

"Almost always? Wouldn't it be always?" Jan seems confused.

"Well, there are cases where medicine attempts to cure a disease other people don't consider to be a disease. There have been attempts to cure diseases like left-handedness, and homosexuality. A cure might not be a favorable outcome for the patient."

"A cure that cures a non-disease. Interesting. You've been thinking about this a lot. It seems Mosbey's has got stuck on a challenging question: does a cure, cure the disease or the patient?" Jan looks up at the clock. "Well, time to get back to work. Maybe if you check a few authoritative medical reference books, you can find a better definition of cure?" They get up and start to clear the table.

"So... none of the medical dictionaries that define cure say cure is to stop a disease?" Jan asks.

"Not only that, one doesn't use the words illness or disease. I

wonder what MERCK says" Jamie replies. *"I'll check tonight. Tomorrow's lunch, then."*

"Tomorrow is my weekend." Jan smiles, *"You've got two days to research. See you Thursday."*

Jan and Jamie have been apart for a few days. Jamie seems more frustrated than ever. As they meet for lunch, Jan opens the conversation.

"So, what does the Merck bible of diagnosis and treatment say about cure?"

"You're not gonna believe this. Merck has no definition for cure. Cure is not in the index, not in the table of contents. The closer I looked, the worse it got."

"How so?" Jan asks.

"Merck is online, so I could easily scan every instance of the word cure in Merck's 11th edition. Cure is not used consistently, and many of the references to cure are cure-rate – a statistical measure of cure, useless in individual cases."

"I can understand that usage might be inconsistent. Merck is written by many authors."

"None of whom appear to use the same definition," Jamie counters, *"I've checked Harrison's Principles of Internal Medicine, Lange's Current Medical Diagnosis and Treatment, and the Diagnostic and Statistical Manual of Mental Disorders (DSM–5). Not one has a definition of cure. Not one lists cure in the index, or the table of contents. Not one makes consistent use of the word cure unless you consider the DSM-5."*

"The DSM-5 is consistent?"

"Absolutely. As near as I can determine, the word cure does not appear at all in the DSM-5." Jamie replies flatly, *"although there is a reference to* **'eventual cures for these conditions**,*' as if we cannot cure any today."*

"So, all mental illnesses are incurable, by lack of definition," Jan laughs.

"So it appears. Actually, the DSM uses words like recovery and remit, even defining partial remission and full remission, but not – as near as I can determine cure."

"Well, to tell the truth," Jan says quietly, *"we don't cure many diseases – to be more honest, most of our patients – we estimate that over 90 percent of our patients recover perfectly well without any need for a doctor. Health cures a common cold, the flu, measles, it heals minor cuts and fractures. We intervene when problems are dangerous, but there are few cases where we can take credit for a cure. When a patient has a chronic disease, it's generally defined as incurable, so even if the patient finds a cure, we call it remission."*

"That reminds me, also checked a Dictionary of Epidemiology, edited by John M. Last, and cure is not in that dictionary either." Jamie commented, and then added, *"and Thomas A. Timmreck, advises in an Introduction to Epidemiology, 'Epidemiology is more interested in prevention and control of diseases than secondary and tertiary curative approaches.'"*

"So, epidemiology the study of causes of disease, ignores cures? Interesting. I'd have thought a cure would prove the cause?"

Jamie replies, with a sad smile. *"It's depressing, isn't it? But on the bright side, I have an idea."*

"You've created your own definition?" Jan looks Jamie directly in the

eyes.

"Yep. I've decided, an illness is cured when the cause has been addressed. Cured is when no more medicines are required for the illness. Healing happens afterwards, if necessary. However, I could not find a single dictionary, or medical reference using the word cause, much less suggesting an illness can be cured by addressing the cause." Jamie laments. *"It's silly."*

Jan thinks for a moment, and then responds *"Healing is a cure, isn't it? And what about surgery? We often use the phrase surgical cure. Although I'm not aware of any test of being cured after a surgery."*

"Modern medicine is suffering from cure blindness," Jamie concludes – as they head out on their rounds.

Jan and Jamie spent only a few days looking for a definition of cure. The conversations are eventually left behind in the day to day hustle and bustle of a hospital job.

Do Medicines Cure?

> Medicine is broken
> *Ben Goldacre, Bad Pharma*

The book **Bad Pharma** contains over 400 pages of *"How drug companies mislead doctors and harm patients."* But almost nothing about cures. The word cure appears less than ten times. Not one is a reference to a medicine or treatment that cures. From the view of Bad Pharma, medicines are treatments of which few, if any, cure.

Cures do exist in medicine, despite their absence in many medical dictionaries and reference texts. Two types of cures recognized by conventional medicine; cures for diseases caused by parasites or pathogens, and surgical cures. Cures for diseases caused by pathogens can be tested and proven, when the pathogen has been eliminated.

Surgical cures have no clear definition of, nor test for cured – the exception being a disease caused by a pathogen, which surgery cures by removing the infected tissue. Most surgical cures cover two other medical conditions – injuries and physical defects.

Medical Cure: Bacterial Infection

The success of medicines like penicillin has led to powerful cure successes and also to a type of medical blindness, medical chauvinism. Bacterial infections are cured by addressing the bacteria that are, the present cause of the illness.

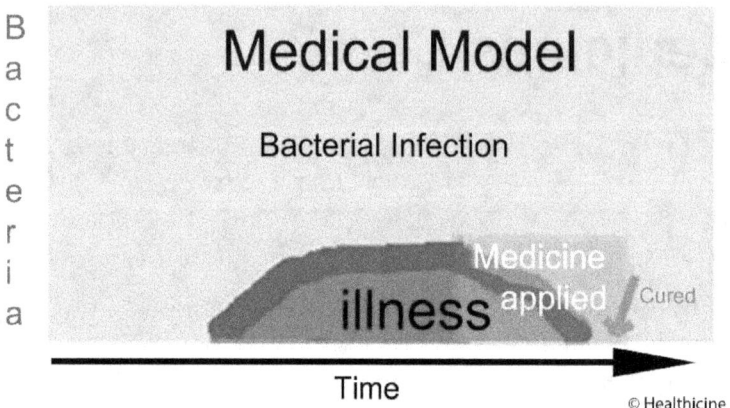

This diagram illustrates curing an illness caused by a pathogen with a medicine. Illness occurs, as the population of pathogen grows.

Medical curing of pathogenic diseases happens in three steps:

- administer the treatment
- allow time for the treatment to work,
- healing.

Verification that the pathogen has been eliminated validates the cure. Healing might be necessary to complete the cure. If the infection regrows, the cure is a failure. A subsequent infection is clearly seen as a new case, not a remission, once a cure has been attained.

The medical model misses many important aspects of cure. As a result, it misses many cures. It is currently impossible to prove a cure of any infection that comes from natural healthy processes – even though this is how most infections are cured. We can understand these issues more clearly, as we explore more comprehensive models of a bacterial infections and their cures.

Medical: Surgical Cure: Bacterial Infection

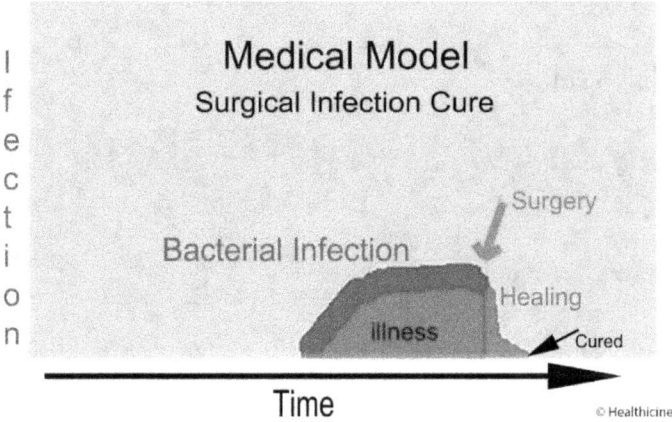

Surgery can also be used to cure a bacterial infection, and the cure can be tested and proven, by demonstrating the bacteria is no longer present. The surgeon cuts out the infected flesh, sometimes cutting off an entire limb or organ. Merck states, for example, *"usually the infected valve must be removed to cure an infection involving the mitral, aortic, or prosthetic valve."*

Important things to note about a surgical cure:

- Surgery is seldom perfect;
- Surgery is only effective for illnesses that are physically localized
- Surgery leaves physical damage, almost always requiring healing to complete the process.
- Surgery generally presents no test for cured, except with infections

The patient might be left with a deficit or disability, but the infection has been cured. The illness is cured, not the entire patient. Cures are not magic, and seldom if ever perfect.

Cure vs Cured

Jan and Jamie are heading to the cafeteria for another lunch. Jamie has been thinking a lot about cure, although they haven't talked about it since their conversation stopped a few months ago. Jamie brings the conversation back to cure.

"I've been thinking a lot about cure these past few weeks," Jamie says quietly.

"Oh, and..." Jan waits for more.

"It's a bit strange," Jamie continues, *"we cure lots of diseases. But we don't pay attention to cures."*

"What do you mean?" Jan turns as they line up their food trays.

*"Well, I had a cold last week, and now I don't have a cold. It's cured. But our medical theories say '**there is no cure for the common cold**.' Isn't that strange?"*

"There is no medical cure for the common cold. The common cold is 'self-resolving.'" Jan explains, *"There are lots of self-resolving diseases: the common cold, the flu, measles."*

"But a disease is not a thing. It's not a self. The common cold has a cause, but the cause is not the disease. So how can it be self-resolving?"

"Well, actually the self that is sick, the health of the patient, resolves the cold." Jan rationalizes.

"But," Jamie continues the argument, *"it's cured."*

"Yes, of course. It was cured by health, by healthiness. And not only that," Jan continues, *"When you are healthier, you cure a common*

cold faster. When you are less healthy, it takes longer."

"That concept works for infectious diseases. Our health fights the infection. But what about non-infectious diseases, like depression? There is no way to tell if depression is cured or just in remission, so depression is generally considered incurable."

"and..." Jan senses that Jamie has more to say.

"But, what if someone's depression is cured? Maybe depression, is curable? How can we know?" Jamie's conversation is bubbling up questions.

"Hmm... Maybe some cases of depression are curable, and some are incurable?"

"Maybe," Jamie asks, *"but how can we tell? Cured is not defined. We can't know if someone has been cured, even if they are cured."*

"Interesting," Jan is thinking. *"we can tell that your cold is cured, even though we don't use the word cured. But we can't tell if a case of depression has been cured. I've never thought about that before."*

Jamie replies cautiously, *"I've been thinking about it a lot. I think the same thing happens with all non-infectious diseases."*

"For example?"

"Well, we've recently declared obesity as a disease. And we can diagnose obesity. But there is no way to diagnosed obesity cured." Jamie waits for a response.

"Well, obesity seems to be a special case. People who lose weight are not necessarily cured. They might go on a diet, and lose weight, and then gain it back over time. They weren't cured, their obesity

was just in remission," Jan counters.

"But, what if, like depression – some patients are cured, and some not cured. We can't tell the difference," Jamie's frustration is showing.

"What does it matter if they're cured?" Jan argues.

"But, if we can't separate cured from remission, we can't get better at finding cures."

"Ok, I can see that." Jan gives a bit, and then presses further, *"are there other examples?"*

"Pretty much any non-infectious disease. Arthritis, scurvy, hypertension, even cancer. We don't diagnose cured for the common cold, measles, and the flu – they are cured by health. And, currently, we can't test or prove cured for any non-infectious disease."

"Interesting. Now that you mention it, I can't think of a single non-infectious disease with a medical test for cured." Jan pauses thoughtfully and concludes with *"Maybe they're all incurable."*

"So, we don't cure diseases? We just treat them? I hope we can do better. I think we can do better. I think we can cure, but we have to take cures and curing seriously first." Jan picks up the tray as they head back to their work in the hospital.

The common cold is cured by health. Healthier people get fewer colds and cure them faster. Influenza appears to be the same. What about depression, obesity, arthritis, even cancer? Can they be cured with healthiness, even when no medicine can cure?

Is health the best medicine? Is health the best cure?

The Process of Curing

As we explore a calculus of curing, we will learn a simple truth: *actions cure.* No medicine is an action. A cure might be a service, but not a product. Unfortunately, conventional medicine, which we might also call we$tern™ medicine, dedicated to dollars, profits, and products, does not believe it possible to profit from curing. Instead, it looks for easier profits from drugs that rarely cure.

> *What then is the cure for hunger? Whatever will allay hunger, that is to say food, and by it the other is cured. Again, drink cures thirst, and moreover, evacuation cures repletion, and repletion evacuation, and rest labour, and labour, rest; and in a word, contraries are the cure of contraries...*
> *And he that does these things best, is the best physician; and he that is most removed from this system is the most removed from a knowledge of the art.*
> *--Hippocrates*

Some diseases are simple, in theory. Scurvy, in theory, is easy to diagnose, easy to cure, and usually easy to tell when the disease has been cured. Unfortunately, few if any medical references recommend a cure for scurvy. Other diseases, like cancer, are difficult to diagnose, difficult to treat – and currently impossible to prove cured. Cancers cured are sometimes counted only after a patient has died from other causes.

Curing is a process. Processes have components, goals, sub-goals, milestones, and end points. Is every disease curable? Is any disease incurable? How can we tell if a disease is curable? With the current definition of disease, it is not possible to prove many cases of disease curable, even after curing them. It is also not possible to prove any case of a disease is incurable; we can only give up the pursuit of a cure.

This book is about curable illnesses. In the interest of brevity and clarity, we will use *"an illness"* to refer to that which is curable, and *"not an illness"* or some other descriptor, for that which is not curable. Therefore, every (curable) illness can be cured. If we judge it cannot be cured, it is not a curable illness and should be called something else, perhaps a disability, a handicap, or even a natural feature.

We need to view each case of disease as consisting of one or more illness components, each of which might be curable, or not. Diseases are often diagnosed via signs and symptoms – without any attempt to isolate causes or curable components. In today's medical practice, there is no concept of a component of a disease, much less a curable component. Epidemiology contains a concept of component causes – but only for prevention, not for curing. Epidemiology is about the flow of diseases through communities, not about individual cases, not about cures. Cure is intentionally not defined in the theory and practice of epidemiology. Every cure is an individual case, not a statistical set.

We need to develop a calculus of curing, a conceptual framework to understand each case of a disease as a set of curable and incurable components. We need to learn to cure components that are curable, and to recognize when they have been cured.

Illness, Disease, Sickness

> *A patient goes to the doctor with an illness,*
> *and goes home with a disease,*
> *Their family sees they are sick.*

What's the difference between an illness, a disease, an ailment, a sickness, a disorder, and many other terms we use for various medical conditions?

The University of Ottawa *"Society, the Individual, and Medicine (SIM) curriculum"* course notes provide a useful perspective to distinguish between illness, disease, and sickness:

"**Illness** *(the person's subjective experience of their symptoms. What the patient brings to the doctor.)*

Disease *(Underlying pathology; biologically defined; the practitioner's perspective. The illness seen in terms of a biological theory of disorder.)*

Sickness *(Social and cultural conceptions of the condition: cultural beliefs and reactions, such as fear or stigma. These affect how the patient reacts, and also what is considered a disorder suitable for medical treatment.)*"

The University of Ottawa statement does not define the reality of an illness, and confuses the medical view with reality. Perhaps sometimes, like blind men examining an elephant, all three perspectives are flawed.

The book **Miracle Cures**, by Robert A. Scott, provides a similar perspective on the difference between disease and illness *"When medical scientists use the term disease, they are referring to what qualified doctors believe is wrong with us; the term illness refers to the patient's subjective experience of the disorder."*

Both the Ottawa document and Robert A. Scott fail to recognize that the doctor's perspective and societies perspectives are also subjective, can change from one doctor to another, from one society or community to another. They fail to notice that the doctor is part of the patient's community. Every diagnosis of a disease is a community perspective.

In this text, I will use the term *illness* to describe the reality of the illness. We must also recognize that every illness has many dimensions, including a physical reality, a mental reality, a spirit reality, and many community realities which include the medical realities.

Perception of an illness changes depending on perspective. Perspectives and perceptions can and should change when treatments are prescribed or administered. The perception of an illness must often change for an illness to be cured. A cure changes – freezes – the perception of an illness, except for speculation about the cause of the cure.

> *If a patient is poor, he is committed to a public hospital as a 'psychotic.' If he can afford a sanitarium, the diagnosis is 'neurasthenia.' If he is wealthy enough to be in his own home under the constant watch of nurses and physicians, he is simply 'an indisposed eccentric.'*
> *- Pierre(-Marie-Félix) Janet*

An Illness

An illness is what the patient has, what the patient is experiencing. An illness affects body, mind, spirits, and community. Illness is a negative concept, although in many cases an illness has positive aspects. It might be a result of positive actions. For an illness to exist, there must be a negative judgment, a judgement that something is wrong. An illness is a problem, in the language of problem analysis, in the book **The New Rational Manager**, *"A problem is the visible effect of a cause."* However, the authors missed a point critical to cure.

A problem is the visible effect of a *present* cause.

There are many different practices and theories of medicine, each with their own theories causes of illness. But they all agree on one thing: Every illness has a cause. Every illness also has negative consequences, the negative effects of the cause.

An illness is not something we can see or touch. An illness is not the opposite of health, an illness is a hole in healthiness.

An Illness is a Hole in Healthiness

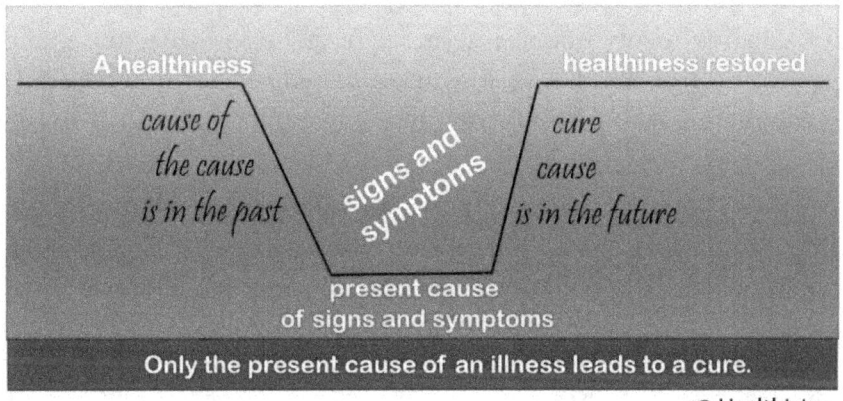

An illness is the intersection of a present cause and its negative consequences, the signs and symptoms of illness. The illness has a chain of causes in the past, which cannot be accessed. The present cause is the cause that can be addressed to produce a cure. The cure is an action, a cause, that addresses the present cause and produces a cure.

An illness is real. The illness to be cured is the illness that exists, which is not necessarily that which is perceived by any observer, including the patient. Curing an illness aligns the reality and the various perceptions.

> *"Every illness can be cured."*
> *- the Healthicine Creed*

From a cure perspective, an illness is that which we believe can be cured.

Neither an illness, nor any case of a disease is a physical thing. We cannot see an illness. We cannot see nor touch a disease. A case of a disease only exists when a medical professional observes a set of signs and symptoms and judges one to be present. A disease, a class of diseases, exists when a community of medical professionals defines a diagnostic protocol for the disease.

A Case of Disease

A disease is formal *"We've got a code for that."* A diagnosis of a disease is a doctor's theory about an illness. A disease is what the doctor diagnoses. An illness begins as a negative judgement by a patient. A disease is an opinion, a judgement, by a medical professional. A case of disease is that which has been diagnosed, a negative judgement by a physician. Diseases and medical conditions are a physician's professional catalog of billable items. However, the concept of a disease is not scientifically defined in medicine. Disease is a statistical concept.

A disease is a concept encompassing many patients with similar illnesses. A while a case of a disease is an individual occurrence of one or more illnesses. In some cases, the cause is clearly defined, and a case of disease is similar or identical to the illness. In other cases, the concept of the disease is based on very little information – such that a case of disease might be diagnosed and treated but cannot be cured and proven cured. Mental disorders, for example, are generally defined without reference to cause, rendering curing and proof of cured impossible.

Classification of Diseases

The ICD10, the International Statistical Classification of Diseases and Related Health Problems is a bureaucratic classification system not a scientific classification. The World Health Organization's page on the ICD purpose and uses claims *"ICD defines the universe of diseases, disorders, injuries and other related health conditions, listed in a comprehensive, hierarchical fashion that allows for: - easy storage, retrieval and analysis of health information for evidenced-based decision-making."* The ICD10 is primarily a statistical and billing tool for medical professionals. A consolidation of *what a doctor (might) diagnose* (disease, medical condition, injury) into a comprehensive list of codes The World Health Organization and the ICD group make no attempt to define disease, much less the *"universe of diseases, disorders, injuries and other related health conditions."* It catalogues codes for billing and encourages medical professionals to use those codes so that statistical data can be collected. It also includes causes and other factors, leading to a list that contains codes for, for example in sequential order:

- W55.21   Bitten by cow
- W55.21XA Bitten by cow, initial encounter
- W55.21XD Bitten by cow, subsequent encounter
- W55.21XS Bitten by cow, sequela (a pathological condition which resulting from a disease, injury, therapy, or trauma, usually chronic)
- W55.22XA Struck by cow, initial encounter
- W55.22XD Struck by cow, subsequent encounter
- W55.22XS Struck by cow, sequela
- W55.29XA Contact with cow initial encounter
- W55.22   Struck by cow
- W55.29XA Other contact with cow, initial encounter
- W55.29XD Other contact with cow, subsequent encounter
- W55.29XS Other contact with cow, sequela

There is no BULL, just COWS, in the ICD10. If a bull gores you, the doctor must choose from the above or a similar list of "other hoof stock" codes, each of which *"describes the circumstance causing an injury, not the nature of the injury."*

A Sickness

Sickness is a judgment by a community. Every individual is a part of many communities throughout their lives. Individuals, their communities, and their relationships to those communities, change continually throughout the lifetime of an individual.

A community might view a person as sick – independent of any illness or disease. When a medical community judges a patient as sick, they are diagnosed with a disease, not a sickness. Sometimes when a patient feels ill, their community views them as sick and provides support. Sometimes the community denies the sickness and refuses to provide treatment. Sometimes a community views a person as sick when no illness or disease is present.

Like an illness and a case of disease, a sickness is not a physical thing. A sickness is an invisible concept that exists when a community judges a person (or perhaps their actions) to be sick.

Illness: That which can be Cured

In summary, the words illness, disease, and sickness are negative judgments of a situation, made by different individuals or communities.

As previously mentioned, in this text, I use the word illness to describe the physical, mental, spirit, or community reality of a medical condition, from cause to consequences, which can be cured.

There are no medical codes for cured. The World Health Organization tracks diseases – but not cures. Even though the ICD10 claims to be *"easy storage, retrieval and analysis of health information for evidenced-based decision-making,"* it cannot be used for decision making about cures.

Mapping Illness to Disease

We often use the word disease and illness interchangeably. An illness and a case of disease are concepts, not things we can see or touch. We can see the signs and symptoms. Sometimes we see or know the cause. To cure any curable illness, we need a clear understanding of illness and the differences between an illness and a disease – which might be curable in whole or in part. Each illness element has a unique cause. Signs and symptoms from a set of causes might be different, similar, overlapping, or identical.

An illness is a specific case in a specific individual at a specific time. Disease, on the other hand, has several meanings. A case of disease can be a specific case. A disease can also be an epidemic, striking many patients over a period of time. A disease can also be the name given to a group of cases of illness with similar signs and symptoms, across many patients - even different species, and across a longer period, even thousands of years.

Causes, even causes of illness, are often present without creating illness. Every illness has a cause. Every cure has a cause. Health has a cause. Diseases, however, are often diagnosed without reference to cause.

A case of illness can be compared to a case of disease, but even this comparison finds many differences. Not every illness is a disease, and not every disease is an illness. The next diagram illustrates differences between an element of illness and a case of disease. It also distinguishes treatments from cures.

A disease is diagnosed by signs and symptoms. Illnesses with overlapping signs and symptoms are often diagnosed as the same disease even when they have different causes.

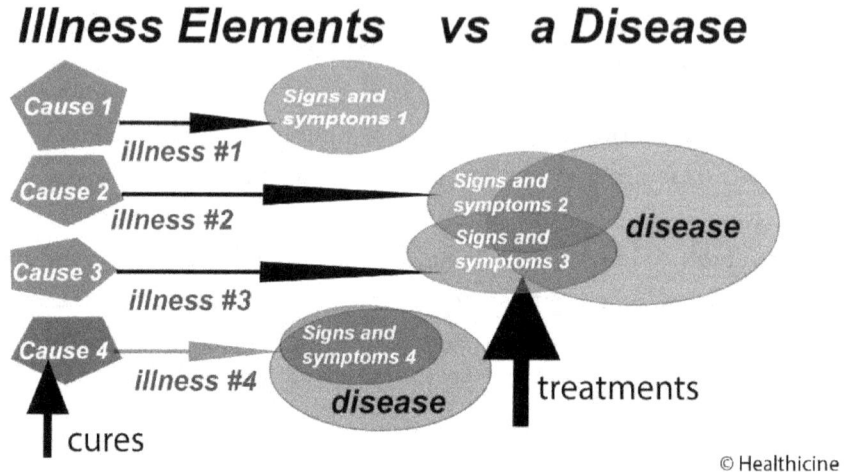

In this diagram, the first disease consists of two illness elements, illness 2 and illness 3 and possibly other factors. The second disease maps closely to illness #4. Disease is often a concept defined and diagnosed without reference to cause, and as a result, many diseases cannot be cured. Disease cures can rarely be tested or proven when they occur. As a consequence, over time most disease cures have come to be considered remission of signs and symptoms.

Treatments for diseases are therefore designed to address or mask the signs and symptoms of a disease – making no attempt to address cause. As a result, most treatments cannot cure. A cure action addresses the cause. As in illness 4, the cause, the link between cause and consequences, and the resulting signs and symptoms fade away as the illness is cured. If the disease maps directly to the illness, it too is cured, but a disease cure is rarely recognized as such.

The definition of a disease is an intentional creation of a threshold of diagnosis. Conventional medicine has an ongoing need for re-definition of each disease to address conflicting risk goals; to catch the disease earlier vs. avoiding dangerous treatments.

When a patient is not ill enough to be diagnosed, or the illness does not match a diagnosis, an illness – and often the patient as well - is often dismissed or ignored. This is an important aspect of the practice of medicine. Many medical treatments are dangerous. They function by reducing healthiness to mask symptoms or by attacking pathogens causing the disease.

Most cures come from healthiness, not from medicines. When we aim to cure, it is important to begin the curing process as early as possible. Increasing healthiness produces cures more effectively and safer than medical treatments, except in emergencies.

The following table illustrates many important differences between an illness and a case of a disease:

An Illness (curable)	A Case of Disease
An illness is what the patient has before, during, and after the diagnosis, until it is cured.	A case of a disease is what is diagnosed.
An illness is a negative condition consisting of a present cause and its negative consequences.	A case of disease is a medical condition with specific signs and symptoms.
Signs and symptoms are only part of an illness. Every illness has a present cause.	Diseases are often diagnosed using signs and symptoms, without reference to any present cause.
An illness is a specific case.	Each "*case of a disease*" is an instance of diagnosis by a physician.
Not every illness is a disease. Many illnesses cannot be and are never diagnosed as a disease.	Not every case of disease is an illness. Many diseases are incurable attributes or disabilities.

A handicap or disability is not a curable illness, although they might be a consequence of illness and a cause of illness.	Codes for and names of diseases include illnesses, injuries, disabilities, signs and symptoms, even some medical tests.
Perception of an illness can vary by patient, doctor, or community, and can change over time.	A case of disease is identified by a doctor, at diagnosis. Other physicians might diagnose differently conditions.

A case of disease can only be cured and proven to be cured, by resolving it into illnesses and curing each in turn. To map a disease to a set of illnesses requires an understanding of causes. Understanding present cause is necessary to cure and to prove any cure.

Conventional medical practice diagnoses cases of disease based on signs and symptoms, which are rarely connected to specific causes. Without awareness of the present cause in each case, the simplest illness cannot be intentionally cured. When cured, even by accident, it is impossible to know or prove it has been cured.

As we study illnesses and cures, we will learn to resolve each case of disease into component illnesses, to determine which can be cured, to find more cures, and better cures, and to know when cures have been accomplished.

Understanding Illness

To understand cure, we need to study illness carefully and thoroughly. Conventional medical experts agree – although seldom explicitly – that most diseases are incurable by medical treatments. But cures exist, and many more are possible. We need to learn to understand cures, and the first step is to understand illness, the general concepts of illness.

An illness is a hole in a healthiness. We each have many, many healthinesses which are constantly changing. Life is to be lived. The active processes of life are constantly exchanging one healthiness for another to move forward. We walk by falling and recovering our balance.

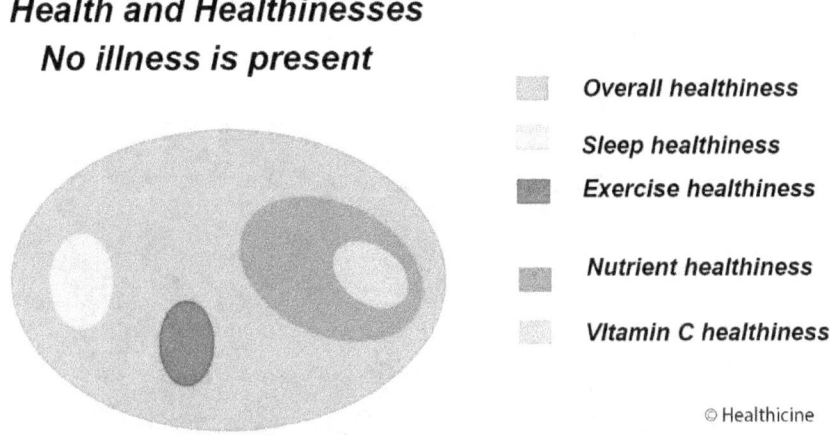

In this diagram, we see a life entity with many different aspects of healthiness. Over time, these healthinesses grow, shrink, and change. Sometimes these changes lead to illness. Some healthinesses are subsets of others. Vitamin C healthiness is a subset of nutrient healthiness.

Over time Vitamin C healthiness might shrink due to a deficiency or absence of Vitamin C in the diet, leading to a Vitamin C deficiency illness which, over time, becomes more severe, and can be diagnosed as the disease scurvy. The illness scurvy creates a hole in the health of the individual. An illness might cause many different signs and symptoms – consequences of the hole in healthiness.

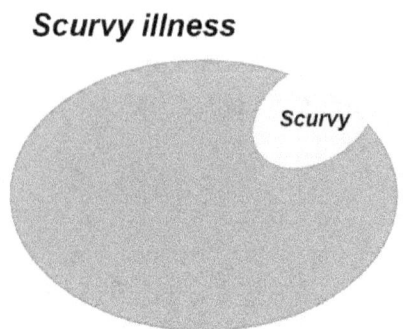

Scurvy illness

Vitamin C deficiency at first is a minor nutrient deficiency. As the deficiency grows over time, it breaks through and becomes the disease:

Scurvy a hole in Vitamin C healthiness

© Healthicine

In this image we see the absence of Vitamin C healthiness creating a hole in the life entity, where health, the essence of life can leak out.

What causes the scurvy?

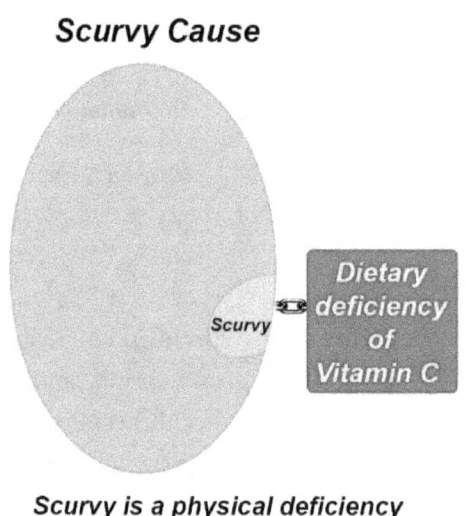

Scurvy Cause

Scurvy is a physical deficiency of Vitamin C, caused by a dietary deficiency of Vitamin C.

© Healthicine

We might think scurvy is *"caused by"* a deficiency of Vitamin C, but that's not an accurate statement.

Scurvy *is* a severe ongoing deficiency of Vitamin C.

The signs and symptoms of scurvy are the signs and symptoms of a deficiency of Vitamin C consumption.

An illness consists of the signs and symptoms and the cause that leads to those signs and symptoms. Every illness has a cause. An illness has another essential component: the link between the cause and the illness, as shown in the above diagram.

An illness is cured by addressing the present cause. The cause is not *a deficiency of Vitamin C.* The deficiency is a cause of the signs and symptoms, but not the cause of the illness. Although many medical treatment texts recommend supplemental Vitamin C for scurvy, it does not cure. Unless the patient's diet is changed, when the supplement, a medicine, is stopped – the scurvy, the Vitamin C deficiency will return. The present illness cause was not addressed.

On the other hand, if the diet is changed, such that it contains sufficient Vitamin C, the scurvy will be cured. Vitamin C as a medicine cannot cure scurvy. Medical treatments are stopped when the illness is cured..

Every illness has a cause. Every cause has a cause. When we begin the analysis of cause, we want to find the *cause of the cause.* Why is the patient's diet deficient in Vitamin C? There are many possibilities.

In the next diagram, we see several potential causes of a cause of scurvy – and in one case, a cause of a cause. Each elementary illness has a single causal chain.

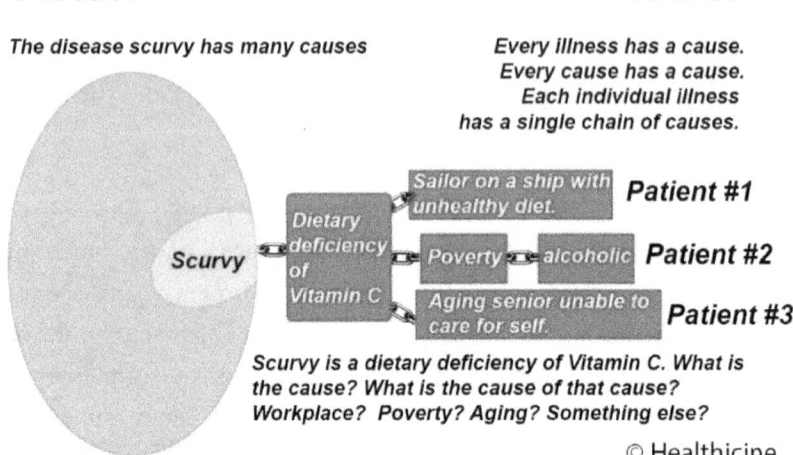

When an illness is caused by a life process, it is cured by addressing the life process on an ongoing basis. Scurvy is almost always caused by a life process.

Illness Causes Illness

As scurvy grows in severity, it causes more illnesses, including injuries and possibly incurable attributes. Conventional medicine names all of the negative consequences signs and symptoms of scurvy. Or does it?

Actually, the illnesses caused by a deficiency of Vitamin C have three or more disease names. At first, it's just a Vitamin C deficiency. Many people suffer deficiencies of Vitamin C for short periods, without any illness. We might suffer a low level, chronic deficiency for a very long period – that is never diagnosed as a disease. Vitamin C deficiency, but not scurvy, is rarely diagnosed. As it becomes stronger, it produces clear signs and symptoms of scurvy, and can be diagnosed and treated. If not treated, it causes further damage to gums, teeth, joints and bones. A dental cavity resulting from scurvy is no longer called scurvy. Further damage that cannot be healed, might be named an incurable disability.

This diagram shows the natural progression of an illness with an ongoing cause, as it is not diagnosed, as it becomes more and more severe.

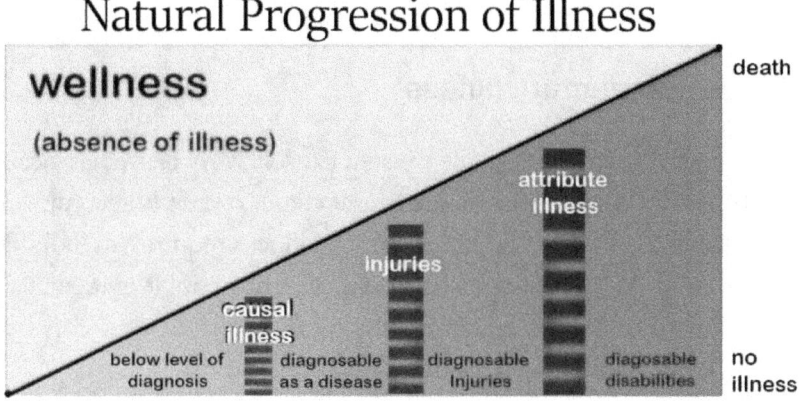

When an illness is caused by a process, like a Vitamin C deficiency, the cure is to address the process cause with a process. These cures are often also preventatives. If the process is not addressed, the illness can lead to injuries.

Injuries are cured by healing. No medicine can cure. Often injuries occur due to causes in the past. The injury is the *present cause* to be cured by healing. When injuries are the result of an illness, there are two present causes – the illness and the injuries. There are two illnesses. Two cures are required.

As an illness progresses to cause damage that cannot be cured, further interventions are necessary to cure. Three or more cures are needed. Conventional medicine sees a single disease and cannot find the *cure*.

When an illness element's present cause a negative attribute that cannot be healed, like a dental cavity, that attribute is the cause. The cure is to transform the negative attribute. Non-surgical transformations are seldom recognized as disease cures. However, cures caused by physical manipulation less invasive than surgery and cures resulting from a transformation of mind, spirits, community or environment are commonplace even though they are routinely ignored by conventional medicine.

Elementary Illness

An element of illness has a single present cause. Every cause has a cause, so an element of illness has a single causal chain. A cure is accomplished by addressing the cause, so each element of illness requires an individual cure. It is possible, perhaps even common, for a single patient to be diagnosed with one disease, with multiple causal chains, thus consisting of multiple elementary illnesses, requiring multiple cures.

With this new understanding, we can make more clarifications and distinctions between an element of illness and a case of disease.

An Element of Illness	A Case of a Disease
An illness element consists of a single present cause or chain of causes and its consequences.	There is no concept of a disease element in today's medical practice.
There are three elementary types of illness: causal, injury, and attribute illnesses.	There is no concept of different disease elements in conventional medicine.
The cause of an illness can exist in body, mind, spirit, community, or environment. Causal chains can link different areas.	Conventional medicine has a poor understanding of cause and causal chains. It also ignores mental, spirit, and community causes.
Causal illnesses have active	Cured is only medically defined for

process causes and are cured by addressing a causal process.	diseases seen to be caused by parasites or pathogens.
Injuries of body, mind, spirit, or community have causes in the past. They are cured by healing the injury, the present cause of signs and symptoms. Healing is a natural cure.	Physical injuries are sometimes diagnosed as diseases, but not injuries to mind, spirit, or community. Although healing is recognized as a type of cure, cured is not medically defined for injuries.
Attribute illnesses are caused by negative attributes of diet, body, mind, spirit, community or environment. Attribute illnesses are cured by transforming the attribute. An injury is an attribute that can be cured by healing.	Diseases caused by negative physical attributes are common, but the concept is poorly studied. Surgery is the only transformation currently considered to cure. Cured is rarely medically testable.
A compound illness has multiple chains of causes resulting in similar or overlapping signs and symptoms. It might consist of several illness elements.	The concept of a compound disease is not defined in conventional medicine. There is no medical nor scientific distinction between a disease with one or more causes.
A complex illness occurs when one illness causes another illness element. Each elementary illness requires a cure.	The concept of a complex disease is not currently defined in medical theory or practice. No known disease requires multiple cures.
A chronic illness has a chronic cause. Causal illnesses are chronic when the cause is chronic. Attribute illnesses are chronic by nature. Injury illness elements are not chronic, because the cause is gone. All	A chronic case of a disease persists over an extended period. There is no understanding of the link between a chronic cause and chronic illness. Chronic diseases are generally

chronic illnesses are attribute illness, cured by addressing the chronic attribute of the cause.	considered incurable.
Every cure is a single case, a cure of a single element of illness. Every cure is a story, an anecdote.	Cured is not defined for most diseases. Anecdotal cures are considered unimportant and unreliable.
By definition: Every (curable) illness element can be cured.	Most diseases can be considered incurable due to the absence of a definition of cured.

A single case of a disease might consist of one or more elements of illness. A case of disease is cured when each component, each illness element has been cured, if possible.

Although an individual illness element might be cured, many diseases cannot be cured due to definitional issues.

Elements of Illness

A single element of illness has a single cause. Each illness element is cured by addressing its cause. Elements that are not curable must be recognized as something other than a curable illness: a disability, an incurable consequence, or perhaps a natural attribute, a feature, or natural consequence of life.

Three Elements of Illness

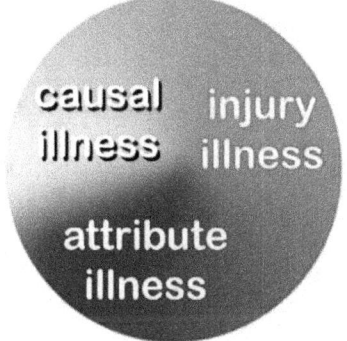

© Healthicine

There are three basic elements of illness.

Causal illnesses are caused by the presence of unhealthy processes or absence of necessary process of diet, body, mind, spirits, or community.

Injury illnesses consist of present damage to the body, mind, spirits, or community, which can be healed.

Attribute illnesses are a consequence the presence or absence of attributes of the patient's diet, body, mind, spirits, community or environment, interfering with life processes.

Most processes are healthy. Many injuries are a healthy part of natural growth process. Most attributes are healthy. The healthy processes of life use attributes to move life forward.

We are familiar with causal illnesses and injury illnesses – but perhaps not so familiar with the concept of an attribute illness. An attribute in itself is not an illness.

Attributes causing illness have causes in the past, like injuries, but they cannot be healed. An injury is a negative attribute that can be healed.

Many attributes are not unhealthy until a situation arises where they cause disruptions and are judged to be negative. We can only move forward in life. Often, changes occur which cannot be reversed. An attribute is a fact, a reality. The negative attribute causing an attribute illness has its own cause, but the illness cannot be cured by addressing that cause. The present illness can only be cured by a change that moves forward – a transformation of the present attribute cause.

There is a gradation between a process cause, an injury cause, and attribute cause of illness. This becomes clear as we work to assign specific causes to an illness. Which cause is the true cause? The cause that leads to a cure.

Life cannot exist without causal processes. Processes act upon attributes and use attributes, creating natural, healthy stresses. Health is present when life processes are moderate, neither excessive nor deficient. Illnesses arise when the stresses of life are extreme or deficient, such that they cause illness or injury. As in this map:

Each type of illness might be caused by a deficiency or an excess.

process deficiency	stress deficiency	attribute deficiency
healthy process	**healthy injury level**	**healthy attribute**
process in excess	excessive stress	attribute excess

© Healthicine

Causal illnesses can be caused by excesses of a process, or a deficiency of process.

Injury illnesses can be caused by an excess of stress, or by a deficiency of stress.

An attribute illness can be a result of the presence of an attribute that interferes with health or a result of the deficiency or absence of attribute necessary to foster healthiness.

Distinguishing Between Illness Types

There are no clear distinctions between the basic elements of illness. Every cause of illness and every cure is a judgment. We make judgements to facilitate curing. A successful cure validates the judgement.

Is depression caused by a dietary deficiency, a process, the loss of a family member or a job, or the stress of a gaslighting spouse? Some cases might be cured simply, others can be more complex and difficult to cure. The cause depends on the cure, is proven by the cure. When we only treat signs and symptoms, even if a cure occurs, we cannot know the cause.

Illness Element

Each element of illness can be viewed as a hole in healthiness.

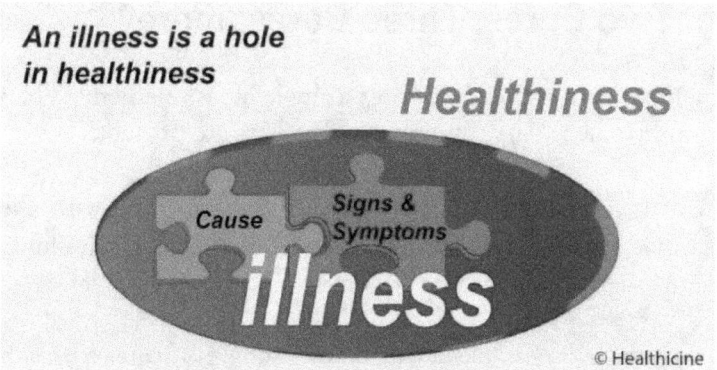

A causal illness is a hole in the health of the patient caused by the presence of an unhealthy process, or absence of a healthy process. An injury illness is a physical hole in the body, mind, spirit, or community. An attribute illness is a hole in ability, caused by the presence of an unhealthy attribute, or the absence of a healthy attribute, a whole – which blocks healthiness.

Each illness element is a puzzle to be solved. The simplistic view that illness is the opposite of health is not useful to cure. An absence of healthiness can grow into to a hole in health, an element of illness.

An illness element is a fundamental unit of illness Each illness element has a single cause and requires a unique cure. Each illness element has:

- a single cause, a single chain of causes and
- a set of consequences, the signs and symptoms of the illness
- an intersection, such that we believe the cause resulted in the consequences.

Each illness element has a single cure, an element of cure.

An illness might be cured by addressing the cause, or by addressing the intersection of the cause and consequences, such that the cause no longer results in negative consequences. Addressing signs and symptoms does not cure.

One Cure, Two Cures, Three Cures, more?

A single elementary cure action cures only a single illness element. When two cure actions are necessary, two illness elements are present.

Don't confuse the concept of *"every illness has a cure"* with the incorrect idea that *"there is only one cure for a disease."* Each illness element presents many opportunities to cure.

Every case of a causal illness has a cause and a chain of causes. Each item in the chain of causes presents opportunities to cure, many opportunities to address the cause. There are many ways to cure any illness. There are many ways to aid the healing of an injury illness, and many ways to transform the cause of an attribute illness.

Once we understand this, we can begin our search for better cures, not just better treatments.

Elements of Cause

Each illness element is a consequence of unhealthiness. There are three basic kinds of unhealthiness: form (attribute), function (process) and when function and form clash (stress).

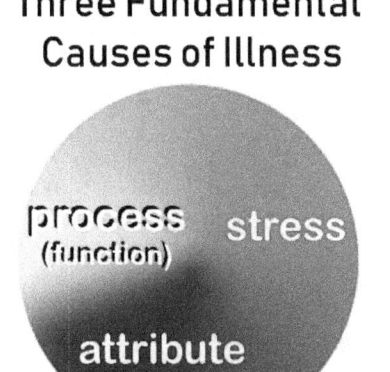

Three Fundamental Causes of Illness

These are the three fundamental causes of illness: unhealthy processes, unhealthy stresses and negative attributes.

Separating the cause from the invisible concept of illness is essential.

The infection illness is not the bacteria, not the bullet, not the dental carie that causes infection.

Illness consists of both the cause and its consequences. Processes, stresses, and attributes are essential to life. They are healthy or unhealthy depending on specific individual circumstances.

A process causes illness when it is deficient or excessive, resulting in a causal illness. A stress is negative when it causes injuries. Stresses that are normally healthy can cause injuries when the stress is severe or deficient, or when healthiness or strength is deficient. An attribute becomes negative or unhealthy when it interferes with, blocks, or leaks healthiness, resulting in an attribute illness.

Causal illnesses often come directly from unhealthiness, from low levels of a healthiness.

Injury illnesses might be caused by healthy or unhealthy actions. They are often caused by other illness or by treatments for diseases.

Attribute illnesses might be caused by natural, healthy or unhealthy actions of life, growth, and aging, even by healing. Many attributes exist and provide valuable functions for years without causing illness until specific conditions arise.

Noun Causes, Verb Causes, Stress Causes

We might ask an obvious question. Are there truly only three fundamental causes of illness – processes, attributes and stresses? Yes. There are three basic causes of illness. This becomes clear when we use more general terms for the three causes.

Process causes are verbs. Attribute causes are nouns. When a verb, a process, interacts with a noun, an attribute, it creates a stress.

Life is a complex web of intentional cause and effect. Physicists often study cause and effect interactions of dead objects, but dead things have no cause, and no effect, they just are. An attribute, a noun, only causes an illness due to an interaction with a live entity. Every causal life event requires a process (a verb) and an attribute the process is interacting with (a noun), which might be another process or attribute. Forces occur in every causal event, healthy or unhealthy. If the force of the interaction is severe enough to cause damage, injuries occur.

We can simplify the three fundamental causes of illness as:

- verb (unhealthy presence or absence of process) causes
- force (unhealthy presence or absence of stress) causes
- noun (negative presence or absence of attribute) causes

Three Causes of Illness

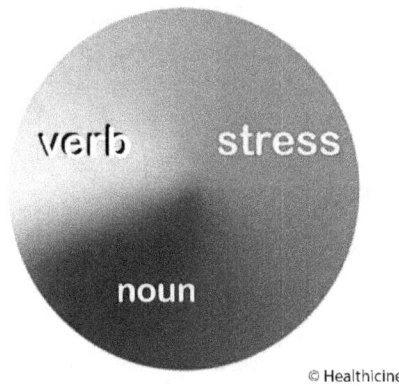

The concepts of nouns, verbs and forces as causes of illness are quite abstract.

In this text will use the more familiar concepts of process causes, attribute causes, and force or stress causes leading to causal illnesses, attribute illnesses, and injuries, respectively.

There are no clear distinctions between processes causes, stress causes, and attribute causes. We make distinctions to facilitate cures.

Diet, Body, Mind, Spirit, Community, and Environment

Today's medical practice locates diseases in the body and ignores cure causes. Most medical treatments address the body, paying little attention to the locations of cause, which limits cure successes.

There are many causes of illness in the body. However, most causes are processes, not things. There are also illnesses with causes in the mind, caused by faulty knowledge, memories, or processing. Some illnesses have causes in the spirits, the intentions and goals, or lack of healthy intentions and lack of healthy goals. Illness are caused by unhealthy communities or unhealthy environments.

Perhaps the most misunderstood word in health today is spirit. The word spirit has many meanings, ranging from emotions, to life spirit, to soul, to spirituality of faith or religion. The word spirit creates fear among medical scientists, who to invoke their own spirit entities, called placebos and placebo effects, for that which they don't understand.

> *In the universe there is an immeasurable, indescribable force which shamans call intent, and absolutely everything that exists in the entire cosmos is attached to intent*
> *-- Carlos Castaneda*

In healthicine, the concept of spirit begins with intention. Spirit, in healthicine, is not about spirituality, not about the soul. That's a question unrelated to cure. Without intention, there is no life. Every living entity has spirits of life, intentions to live – or it dies. Many social animals, like dogs and humans, are very good at discerning intention in others – although often confused or mistaken as well. Sometimes we deliberately misrepresent our intentions for personal benefit. We don't just have spirits, we make conscious and unconscious use of them throughout our daily lives, for the health of it.

Without intention, there is life, no health, no illness, and no cures. Every life entity has many intentions, many spirits. A single cell has intentions to survive, to live, to grow, and to reproduce by division. A species, a genetic line of cells has intentions to evolve, to adapt to their environment as it changes as it evolves, to survive as a species or adapt and change in order to survive. Individual cells have intentions to compete, to defend themselves, and to cooperate, to help each other.

The intentions, the spirits of individuals are competitive, those of the community are cooperative. Each individual lives in many communities. The distinction between individual and community, between competition and cooperation, is never perfectly clear.

> *The gene is the basic unit of selfishness.*
> *--- Richard Dawkins, The Selfish Gene*

Richard Dawkins failed to notice that for to selfishness to exist, a community of cooperation is required. Individual life entities, and even genes are not strictly selfish, nor strictly altruistic. Life persists and advances when competition and cooperation are combined and coordinated to move forward in life. Genetic components compete and cooperate to survive, reproduce, and evolve. Because genetic components are not alive, we might say they don't have spirits – but when they work in cooperation to create a living cell, spirits emerge and become an essential aspect of life. Cooperation is a powerful spirit, emerging without intention. Cooperation creates success. Successful life entities find more cooperation. The duality and harmony of competition and cooperation is the essence of life. Competition cannot exist without community, and community does not exist without cooperation. Genes are not alive as individuals, but their spirits live on in their communities, creating life and persisting as components of life entities.

As we study the hierarchy of healthicine, from genetics and nutrients to cells, tissues, limbs and organs, organ systems, complex bodies, minds, spirits, and communities – we find spirits in each layer. Spirits, intentions of individuality, of competition, and spirits of community, of cooperation, are essential to the hierarchies of life. The entire hierarchy is a living balance between spirits of competition and cooperation. Individuals compete. Every individual lives in a community. As soon as an individual reproduces, it creates and becomes part of a community which benefits from cooperation. Cell lines and cellular communities establish their individuality and find individual success by competing with other cell lines and communities – and find higher levels of success by cooperating within their community and with other communities. When cells and cell lines cooperate, they form tissues that evolve in cooperation. Limbs and organs evolve as tissues cooperate for the benefit of a higher-level body. Limbs and organs also compete. If one gets more work, or more nutrients, it grows larger and demands more again.

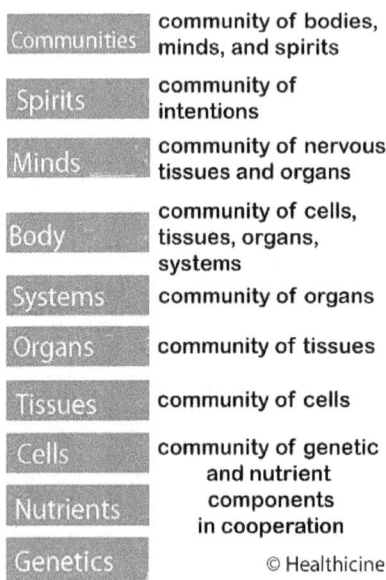

Communities	community of bodies, minds, and spirits
Spirits	community of intentions
Minds	community of nervous tissues and organs
Body	community of cells, tissues, organs, systems
Systems	community of organs
Organs	community of tissues
Tissues	community of cells
Cells	community of genetic and nutrient components in cooperation
Nutrients	
Genetics	© Healthicine

Each step up the hierarchy of healthicine, from genetics to cells, to tissues, to organs, to body, mind, spirit and communities of individuals, comes not from individuals, but from the cooperation of individuals that forms the next community, the entities at the next layer.

Each successful community reproduces to create a new layer of individuals, with new spirits, new intentions of competitiveness and new opportunities to cooperate.

Humans begin life as a single cell, that multiplies into a cooperating cellular mass, which then segregates into cooperating tissues, and develops into cooperating organs, limbs and organ systems to form the body. When a baby exits the womb, they merge with and begin to cooperate with other life entities, from family and friends to bacteria, fungi and viruses in their environment. Every individual human consists of many individual cells and tissues, competing and cooperating, each with spirits of individuality and spirits of cooperation that create the body. That first cell needs powerful spirits to develop into a human, or it fails. The cellular mass expands these spirits, these intentions. Tissues, limbs, organs, and organ systems develop their own spirits, expand, enhance and become part of the spirits of life in every human. Each individual becomes part of the spirit community of humans. When an individual spirits of life fades, the individual fades and dies, but the community persists and evolves, creating new individuals and new communities. The intentions, the spirits, persist.

In the current scientific models of biology and medicine, spirits don't exist. Medicine studies individuals and ignores non-physical attributes, including communities – until those communities become strong enough to create a new level of individuals. Spirit is non-physical, so it is ignored, actively shunned by current sciences of life. As a result, we fail to understand the spirits of health and healthiness, and we fail to understand cure.

The body is the individual in the hierarchy of life. Body refers to the physical aspects and physical processes of an individual life entity. The body refers to anatomy, the study of body parts, and their functions. In the hierarchy diagram, we position body above cells, tissues, organs, and organ systems. But, every life entity, from cells to trees, to humans, has a body. Every cell in our human bodies is an individual cell, and also has a body.

Mind relates to the attributes and processes of memory, calculation, and learning. The body is a whole, more than the sum of the parts. The mind is not a physical entity. The mind is a whole, more than a sum of attributes, functions and processes. Mind is separate from physical attributes and processes, even though it disappears when the body stops functioning. It is a whole, separate from the brain and body. The mind does not exist solely in the brain. When we practice a sport, for example, we teach our limbs to coordinate their activities. When we change our diet, or even the timing of consumption, we teach our bodies to respond to the new diet – sometimes even leading to genetic changes. Every single-celled animal has a mind, consisting of the lessons it has learned from its current life, and those it has learned and remembers from past lives, through genetics and structure.

In the hierarchy, we place mind above the body, but every life entity, and every component has a mind. There is a hierarchy of mind, from cells to tissues, to organs, organ systems, and body. Even spirit and community have elements, attributes, and processes of mind. Humans also have mind, or mental components that come from our history, from our genetics, and mental components that are learned. We extend our minds with life and art. Art is an extension of the mind, spirits, and community.

Spirit consists of senses, emotions, intentions, motivations, goals, passions, and drive. Every individual life form has life spirits, or it dies.

In the hierarchy, we typically position spirit above the mind, perhaps because it is more mysterious. But like mind, every life entity has spirits of life. Every cell, every tissue, organ, organ system, body, mind, and community has spirits to persist, to grow, to reproduce and to evolve.

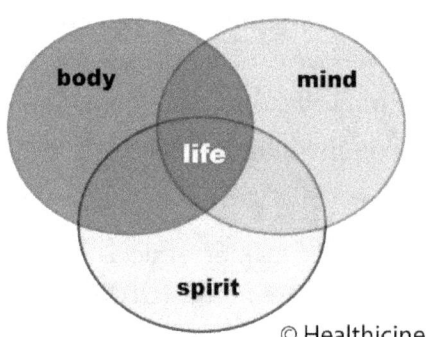

We often see body, mind, and spirit represented as a set of overlapping circles. Religions and other philosophies sometimes represent soul as the intersection in the centre.

Life does not exist without all three.

All three, body, mind, and spirit must be present in cooperation, in community, to create a living entity. If any fails, the individual life ends. Each is a hierarchy created by and consisting of many layers in the hierarchies of life and health.

When our spirits are low, we might feel dead or wish we were dead. Every living cell also has spirits, intentions to live, to grow, to eat, to excrete, and to reproduce. Tissues, limb and organs, bodily systems, and bodies each have spirits – goals and intentions - at their level. Humans and many animals have spirits at higher levels: mental spirits, life spirits, individual id and ego spirits, community and cultural spirits. Individual humans have a super-ego, a community component of their individual spirits. Spirits are the intentions of a life entity or a community, which constantly seek and use balances, competition, and cooperation to individual and community advantage.

Communities are essential to any life entity. No living cell can survive on its own. As soon as a cell multiplies it becomes a community. Humans extend the concept of communities to the creation of communities that grow, persist, and evolve for thousands of years. We write down our thoughts and ideas. A person, or a community in the present, can use the concepts and ideas written down thousands of years ago, or yesterday, and ideas that look far into the future.

Environment is also many layered. Tissues are environments for cells; organs are environments for tissues; the body is an environment for an organ. The air we breathe constitutes an environment of our lungs. Our communities are an environment for our minds and spirits.

This table presents a comprehensive view of causes of illness by type of cause mapped against the environmental layer in the hierarchy of body, mind, spirit, and community:

Source of Cause	Causal Illnesses is Caused by:	Injury Illnesses is Caused by:	Attribute Illnesses is Caused by:
Body	Physical Processes	Force or stress of Body	A Physical Attribute
Mind	Mental Processes	Force or stress of the Mind	A Mental Attribute
Spirits	Spirit Processes	Force or stress of Spirits	A Spirit Attribute
Communities	Community processes	Force or stress of Community	A Community Attribute
Environments Internal or external	Processes of Environment	Force or stress of the Environment	An Attribute of Environment

When we locate a cause in diet, body, mind, spirits, communities, or an external environment, we are making a judgement. The boundaries between these layers are not clear distinctions. We make judgements to facilitate curing.

An illness is a disruption. Signs and symptoms of an illness can affect the entire hierarchy of body, mind, spirit, community, and environment. We identify the cause of an illness element to facilitate curing. A cure attempt is a test of a causal hypothesis.

The Intersection of Cause and Consequences

Illnesses have another important component that can lead to cures. Illness occurs when an intersection of cause and consequences are judged to cause to illness.

We can view an illness element as having four three parts:

- the subject; the present cause,
- the objects; one or more healthinesses affected by the cause,
- the intersection; such that we believe the cause responsible for the consequences
- the signs and symptoms of illness.

Components of an Illness Element

Effects: the signs and symptoms of illness
present cause — intersection → healthinesses affected

© Healthicine

The consequences of a cause, the signs and symptoms of an illness, are dependent on the strength of the cause, the healthiness of the patient, and their intersection. The strength and duration of a cause can often be measured objectively. The strength and healthiness of a life entity might also be measured as it relates to a cause. We often ignore the intersection.

This model provides three opportunities to cure any illness. We might address the causal chain, or improve the patient's healthiness, or break the link between the causal chain and the patient's illness. Addressing the signs and symptoms cannot cure.

For example: a person might suffer from a deficiency of Omega 3 nutrients, because they don't like fish. We can try to change their dislike for fish, or force or trick them into eating fish. Those actions might cure. Or, we might deflect the cause, providing other foods that contain Omega 3 nutrients, breaking the link between disliking fish and illness, and cure by improving the patient's healthiness.

Proof of Cause

A cure proves the cause of an illness. There is no stronger proof of cause, no other proof of cause. Proof by prevention identifies statistical causes, seldom useful to cure present cases of illness. All illnesses have causes in the present. Intentional curing of a present illness proves the present cause.

Does smoking cause cancer? Maybe. Smoking is part of a long causal chain that does not necessarily lead to cancer. Smoking causes cancer statistically. But everything causes cancer statistically. Smoking, however, does cause smoker's cough. This is proven when stopping smoking cures smoker's cough. But, if the cure is delayed, the illness might become an incurable attribute, a disability like chronic incurable bronchitis, or COPD (Chronic Obstructive Pulmonary Disease).

A cure is an action, a cause that brings about a cure of an illness, proving the cause of the illness. Of course, proof by cure might be wrong – other factors might have brought about the cure. But, right or wrong, if we wish to find cures, we must search for them.

Statistics about non-cures, about treatments providing benefits to a patient's signs and symptoms, tell us nothing about cures. Such statistics can, all too easily, direct our attention away from actual cures. Statistical cures, like *cure rate,* are bureaucratic measures that do not represent, much less prove cured in any specific case. Only statistics of cures can support evidence of a successful cure.

Cure Cause

A cure cause is an illness cause which, when addressed, produces a cure element. The action addressing a cure cause is the cause of a cure.

Causal Chains

Every illness has a cause. Every cause has a cause. Causal chains can link to and from diet, body, mind, spirit, community, and environment. Depressed spirits might lead to lack of physical or mental exercise, to a faulty diet, to decreased healthiness and increased frequency of injury.

What is a cure cause? A cure cause of an illness, is a *present cause* which when successfully addressed, cures the illness. When we say the cause of a present illness "was" something, we are referencing a past cause. This is appropriate to identify the cause of an injury of an attribute, but does not identify a present cause, and cannot identify a cure cause. Addressing past or future causes cannot cure unless the cause is also present.

It is important when studying the concept of cause to recognize that causes don't just cause illness. There are causes of healthiness as well as causes of cures.

Every cause of illness has a cause. Every illness element has a unique chain of causes. There are causes in the present and causes in the past. To cure, we must address a present cause. Causes in the past are hypothetical and cannot be proven, cannot be used to produce a cure unless they are also present. When there is a single causal chain, addressing any cause will break the chain and cure the illness.

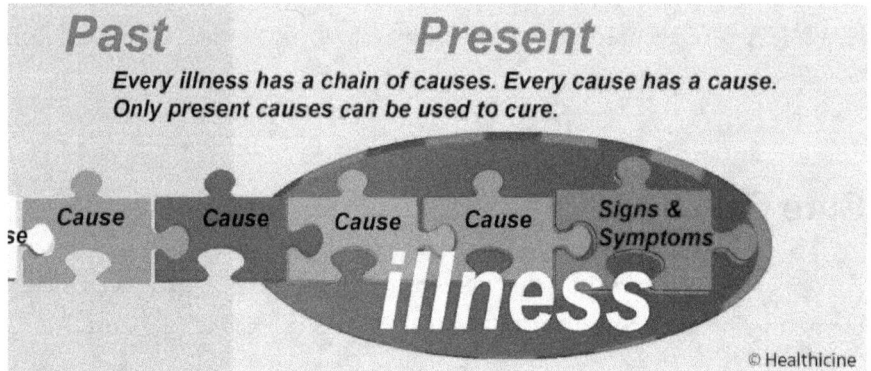

The chain of past causes might be expanded forever. When we research the chain of causes, we are often able to extend the chain of causes in both directions from any identified cause. Causes are fractal, we can zoom in closer and closer to each cause and see smaller causal components. The length of a causal chain is limited only by our understanding and our imagination.

We can explore chains of causes with questions:

What is the cause of this cause?

What is caused by this cause?

Often, a link in the chain of causes is present because it provides a benefit to the patient. This is especially true for chronic illnesses. It is important to ask, for every present cause in the chain:

How am I benefiting from this cause?

This is often a question the patient must ask themselves. When a physician asks, there may be disbelief, denial, and resistance.

We ask these three questions again and again as our understanding grows closer to finding a cure.

Causal illnesses chains have ongoing process causes in the present. A true process causal chain is such that a process which successfully addressing any link in the chain results in a cure of that illness element. We cannot prove a hypothetical link in a chain until addressing one results in a cure. Every cure attempt provides new information, even if it fails to cure, that can be used to understand more, and to continue the quest for a cure.

Injury illnesses have causes in the past, and causal chains in the past. Addressing a cause might prevent future illnesses but cannot cure a present injury. The injury itself is the present cause of the negative signs and symptoms. The cure is to heal the injury, a natural transformation.

Attribute causes also have causes in the past, which might be used to prevent illness, but cannot cure. A negative attribute typically causes illness by disrupting, blocking or leaking a healthy flow or activity. Attribute illnesses are cured by a change, by transforming the attribute, the present cause. Sometimes a cure of an attribute illness occurs through a transformation of perception of the negativity of the illness. These too are real cures, not placebo effects.

Because the causes of an attribute cause are in the past, the present portion of a process causal chain ends when an attribute cause is identified.

In some cases, it is most effective to search for an attribute cause to produce a cure, because process cures require ongoing processes – while attribute causes need only be addressed once. However, this approach can sometimes lead to false causes and false cures. A patient with a chronic infection illness might be treated with an antibiotic that kills the infection attribute but does not address the chronic cause of the infection. What appears to produce an attribute cure fails to address the higher-level cause. The chronic illness might only be cured by attention to cleanliness, a lifelong process commitment.

Sometimes, the distinction between a process cause and its cure, and an attribute cause and its cure is less distinct. A chronic repetitive stress illness like carpal tunnel syndrome might be cured by a change in working posture – a process – or it might be cured by a new chair – an attribute – that forces a change in posture.

When there is more than one causal chain, there exists more than one illness element. Sometimes a causal chain splits into two chains. In this situation, a single cure might be possible at one point in the chain, but if addressed at a different point in the chain, two cures are necessary. An illness is a single illness element when one action cures, and two illnesses when two cures are required. Finding a different cure element can re-define the illness by refining our understanding of the cause and the causal chain.

Duality of Cause

The concepts of cause and effect present a complex problem to philosophers and physicists, who have debated for centuries even about their existence. In physics, cause and effect generally refers to two linked events or processes, the cause – in the past, and the effect – in the future with respect to the cause. In the philosophy of causality, a bumblebee cannot cause itself to fly. But bumblebees don't study philosophy or physics. They intend to fly, and they fly in the present, pushing the hypothetical causes into the past. Even at the levels of physics and philosophy, the concept of cause and effect requires life. Only life forms make definitions of X and Y, and judgements of cause. Without life, things happen, but without need or ability to define cause and effect.

Cause and effect are simpler when we study life, healthiness, and illness. Life, living entities, use cause and effect to survive, to grow, to reproduce and to evolve. Life is a chain of intentional causes and effects that cannot exist without cause and effect. Life creates and uses cause and effect to serve life, to cause healthiness. Most causal processes do not cause illness.

Life, healthiness, and illness are processes, not events. Causes of healthiness and causes of illness are present and active, interacting with other active processes. The cause of a causal illness part of a life process. Life is a constant flow of processes. Sometimes the flow is disrupted, leading to illness. Every single disruption has a cause.

To cure illness, we must focus our attention on cause. At the same time, we must be aware that every illness is a judgement. Every illness has a cause, and every cause is also a judgement.

For a cause to have an effect, it must affect something. Cause and effect have a dual nature requiring a subject (the cause) an object (the affected) and their intersection in time.

Causes of illness have effects on the healthiness a life form. Every time we identify a specific cause of an illness, we must attend to the duality of cause.

We often focus our attention on one side, the cause, and don't notice the other side, the healthiness that counters the cause. We naturally see negative causes as coming from outside. Focus is important. It brings clarity and helps us get results.

However, ignoring the duality of cause can miss many cures.

The Duality of Cause

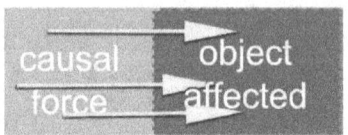 =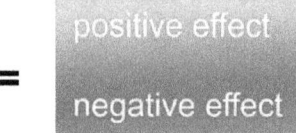

The effect of a cause depends on its strength and on the strength of the object being affected.

Judgement links cause to consequences and evaluates them as positive or negative.

© Healthicine

To cure, and to study curing, we isolate individual causes. But we must not limit our view to individual effects. In life, every cause can have many effects. Every live form consists of body, mind, spirits, and community. Every cause might have positive and negative effects on body, mind, spirits, and community. Healthiness consists of the totality of diet, body, mind, spirits, and community. Sometimes we observe an illness in a single area – most often in the body. Other illnesses, like dementia, have their strongest effects on the mind – although conventional medicine often places these effects in the brain. Depression is a strong effect on the spirits – a serious challenge for conventional medicine, which fails to recognize the concept of spirits. Violence a strong effect on the community aspects of the patient or sometimes of the community on the patient.

Cause is reductionistic. We isolate causes to produce cures, to meet cure goals.

Consequences are holistic.

Most of the time, when we encounter causal forces, they don't cause illness. Our healthiness naturally makes use of cause and effect to move life forward. Our bodies, minds, spirits, and communities have many healthy abilities to make use of causes, to deal with cause and effect, and if necessary, to deflect causes, to adjust for causes, to avoid negative consequences from potential causes of illness.

Cause: Stronger Causal Force

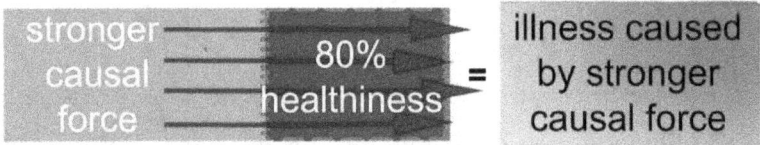

Stronger causal forces can cause illness, even in individuals with very healthy bodies, minds, spirits, and communities. © Healthicine

Sometimes the cause of an illness is stronger than a healthiness. Illness occurs. While a cause continues to be present and continues to be stronger than our healthiness, illness continues, sometimes it grows and causes healthiness to shrink.

Healthiness Cause

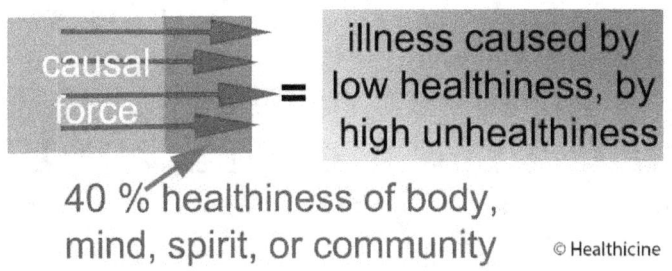

40 % healthiness of body, mind, spirit, or community © Healthicine

In this diagram, a healthiness is low, and a weaker causal force, possibly one normally present in the patient's internal or external environment, might cause an illness. In cases like this, the cause of the illness might be less clear, difficult to discern. When an illness is due to a causal force which normally would not cause illness – we can judge the cause to be a lack of healthiness.

How can we know the true cause of an illness? There might be many theories, but the solution is trivial. We identify a true cause by curing. If we address a specific cause and addressing it cures the illness, that was the cause. We might argue there were multiple causes, but the illness has been cured. Theoretical causes might be important for prevention, but they can no longer cure.

Are there illness elements that have two causes? No. By definition: if a single action cures, it was a single illness element, if it requires two actions to cure, there were two illness elements. The cure defines the cause.

An illness caused by a slightly stronger causal force and a slightly weaker patient healthiness is a single illness element when addressing any single cause results in a cure. Of course, a cure might have come from natural healthiness, from healthy processes, regardless of conscious attempts to understand cause, regardless of our attempts to cure. The common cold, the flu, and measles are commonly cured without conscious intent.

When we believe there are two or more causes of a specific illness, we might address all of them at once – or two, or only one. Whatever actions we decide to take might cure, or not. Once a cure is present, we can no longer identify the cause – unless we recreate the illness, by recreating a cause. Proof of cause is of little importance to a cured patient.

Addressing many causes at once increases the likelihood of a cure. We might remove or reduce several negative causal forces and also improve healthiness. Identifying a specific cause is only accomplished by using addressing one potential cause at a time. However, this can be a slow, time consuming, error-prone process. Even when it cures, we can't be certain we have addressed the cause. Every illness exists in a living, breathing, growing, aging entity. Many potential causes of illness are changing at once. A more effective approach is to improve many aspects of healthiness at once, which cures faster. The side effects being improved healthiness.

Every Cure has a Cause

Every cure element has a single cause. People in primitive societies believe illnesses are caused by evil spirits or evil beings beyond our control, and cures are caused by good spirits, miracles, or the actions of saints. Today we use the names *placebo* and *placebo effect* for that which we do not understand. It's a similar error. Don't be distracted by the mysticism of placebo effects. A placebo effect is an effect we don't understand, with a real cause, a real chain of causes. As soon as we understand, it's no longer a placebo effect. Placebo effects are rarely cures, and when they are – the cure is not likely to be recognized or acknowledged. Placebo cure is not in the dictionary.

If we attempt to address the cause of an active illness element, and it does not cure the illness, either we have not yet successfully addressed the identified cause, or it was not the cause of the illness element.

Two different illnesses, one caused by an external force, and another caused by internal unhealthiness, might often be diagnosed as a single disease. Diagnosis seldom identifies specific causes. An illness with by two different causes requires two cure actions. Cures prove cause. Multiple cures prove multiple causes.

If a patient has a bacterial infection due to a cut it is usually cured naturally, by natural healthiness. The cause is gone. If not, an antibiotic might cure it, addressing the bacterial cause, while the body heals. On the other hand, if a patient has a bacterial infection because of an unhealthy work environment, curing with an antibiotic is a treatment that provides only a temporary benefit. The cause has not been addressed.

The treatment only addressed the infection, the current signs and symptoms, but not its present cause.

A person with many healthinesses far below a healthy level, who suffers more illnesses caused by minor stresses, is less healthy, not just unlucky. Someone who suffers more illnesses than normal because of sporting activities should sometimes be judged *less healthy* overall than someone who is not so strong, but takes fewer risks.

Every cause of every illness has this dual potential. Each cause can lead to illness when it is stronger than the health of a life entity and will not cause illness if the causal force is below the strength of the person's healthiness. This is obvious when we work to cure illnesses. Mysterious when we treat diseases with no intention to cure.

Mind and Spirit Duality of Cause

Causes of illness are not just physical. Many causes of illness come from our mind, from incorrect knowledge, incorrect calculation or planning. Many illnesses are caused by unhealthy spirits, driving us towards unhealthy activities, or away from healthy activities. Many injuries and other illnesses are caused by unhealthy communities.

Mind and spirit causes also have duality. A weaker cause has a larger effect on a weaker patient. The consequences can also affect body, mind, spirits, and community. Consequences are holistic. When we believe, in our mind, that the cause is stronger than us, it can have a stronger effect. When we believe we are stronger, we will tolerate more severe symptoms, and fight harder. When our spirits, our intentions are to fight the illness, to survive, a cause will have less effect, be less likely to cause illness and will cause illnesses that are less severe. The strength of our communities has a similar effect. If our communities give up, we might give up. When they fight harder, they help us to fight harder. Improving healthiness and strength of mind and spirits and communities are valuable curative techniques.

We need to study and learn to make use of, not just the physical duality of cause, but also the mind and spirit dualities of cause. Anything less is unscientific and insufficient.

Duality of Each Cause in a Causal Chain

Every present link in a causal chain has a dual nature. At every link in the chain, the consequences of the cause depend on the strength of the cause, the intersection, and the strength of the healthiness of the life entity subjected to the cause. We rarely measure the strength of the link. It is usually attributed to the cause.

The strength of past and future causes is important to evaluation of past illnesses and the prevention of future illnesses, but cannot be used to cure.

Active Chronic Causes: Habits and Routines

Many life entities form habits and routines to save time and energy, and to bring consistency to their lives. Humans are unique in that we can think consciously about our habits and routines, sometimes even giving them names. We have a conscious ability to adopt habits and to change our habits. Habits and routines might also develop and change without conscious intent, sometimes with negative consequences. Habits and routines can increase or decrease healthiness; they can cause, or cure illnesses. We often viewed habits as causing illness. Charles Duhigg, author of The Power of Habit, says that individuals have habits, while communities have routines. With this distinction we might cure many individual illnesses by addressing or creating a habit, and many community illnesses by addressing or creating a routine.

A habit might be viewed as an attribute of the patient, or as a life process. Duhigg advises that transforming a habit is generally easier than trying to create a new habit or get rid of an older one.

A healthy habit, such as walking a mile every morning, might bring dramatic improvements in health, for people who are not active enough. On the other hand, it might produce injuries in someone who is weak, sick, or enfeebled.

In individual circumstances, smoking might lead to temporary health benefits, but over time a habit of frequent smoking can have serious negative effects on healthiness.

> *The problem is that there isn't one formula for changing habits. There are thousands.*
> *- Charles Duhigg. The Power of Habit*

Many unhealthy habits can be transformed into healthy habits, or be replaced by a healthier habit. Sometimes, we can simply stop an unhealthy habit – but that can be very difficult.

> *To cease smoking is the easiest thing I ever did. I ought to know because I've done it a thousand times. —*
> *attributed to Mark Twain and others*

There are many cures for any illness caused by an unhealthy habit.

The Dishrag Cure

In 1979, I was smoking a lot of cigarettes and wanted to quit. I needed to address my smoking habit, and the method I chose was unique. As I tapered off to fewer and fewer cigarettes, I made the following simple rule for myself.

First, I removed all ashtrays, but one, from the house. If I wanted to smoke, I had to go to the kitchen cupboard and get that ashtray. Then, I could have a cigarette. After I had my cigarette, I washed the ashtray, dried it, and put it away.

Before long, smoking became a filthy chore. This new habit helped me to smoke less and less, and I soon quit completely. We still have the ashtray – for when friends visit. We let them use it on the balcony and wash it after they leave.

Trigger Causes

The concept of a trigger is frequently used in medicine although it is poorly and inconsistently defined. A trigger suggests an image of a gun. A small pull on the trigger releases a huge force: like a bullet causing a lot of damage. However, in conventional medicine, a trigger can mean many different things. An infection might be seen as triggered by an injury, even a small scratch. In some cases, conventional medicine views stressful events as triggers – if they are followed by a chronic disease -- as if the stressful event pulled a trigger. This mistake is easily made when chronic diseases are viewed as incurable.

Triggers are often described as *"the straw that broke the camel's back,"* but triggers are rarely the cure cause of an illness. When an illness is present, the trigger is in the past and cannot be accessed to cure.

In the healthicine model, a trigger is a stress that pushes a person over a breaking point. The trigger's action is the final breakdown of a defense that has been maintained for some time.

When a person has an unhealthiness, causing minor damage, invisible danger can creep higher and higher. At some point, it reaches a threshold, and suddenly a small change appears to trigger a catastrophe – like the trigger of a gun.

Trigger Causes Release an Overloaded Unhealthiness.

One cause is creating an unhealthiness just below an illness threshold. The trigger releases the unhealthiness, appearing to cause the illness.

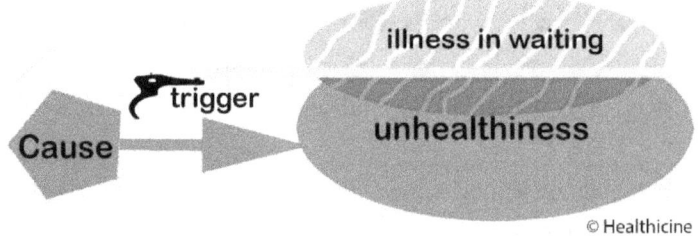

A triggered illness has two parts: an *illness in waiting* or *in remission* and an event, possibly a minor illness, sometimes even a healthy action, that releases the pressure of the illness in waiting.

The hidden illness is the large unhealthiness, held at bay by other healthy forces, not yet judged to be an illness, not yet diagnosed as a disease. When a significant unhealthiness exists, there is always danger it will cross some threshold or that some trigger event will release the pressure. The trigger has little effect when no healthiness is overloaded. The concept of a trigger is often important in mental illness, where a specific thought or action can release the built-up pressure of negative thoughts, emotions, or spirits.

It's easy to mistake the trigger for the cause of an illness or injury which must be healed while the trigger disappears. Once the trigger releases and the patient recovers from the pressure release, the signs and symptoms might be suppressed by future actions, giving the impression of a cure. Treating signs and symptoms once the trigger has fired does not cure the underlying illness. The result is usually an ineffective, temporary cure.

There are two ways to cure a trigger illness. When we view the presence of a trigger as an attribute cause, we can aim for a cure by avoiding or transforming the trigger. Many people learn to avoid a trigger. However, avoiding the trigger does not address the unhealthiness. It is always possible that another trigger will emerge, or that the illness will emerge without a clear trigger. Someone who has severe anger, panic, or depression in response to a trigger might address one trigger only to find another emerge. The trigger is rarely the cure cause.

The best cure is to improve healthiness, to address the present cause of the underlying illness. This cure might be invisible when the underlying illness is not visible, and only become apparent over time, when the trigger fails to cause another instance of illness. Proving that the hidden illness is cured is difficult, requiring strong confidence in the cause and that it has been addressed.

Composite Illnesses

A single illness element, an elementary illness, has a single present cause, many negative consequences, and a single cure.

Elementary Illness

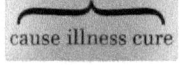 An **element of illness** has a single present cause. It persists until the cause is addressed, and the signs and symptoms have faded and gone. The illness element has been cured.

Every **illness element** has a present cause. The illness progresses until the cause is addressed. Past causes cannot be accessed to cure.

An **illness** has negative signs and symptoms due to the cause.

A **cure** reverses the present cause. Signs and symptoms fade and disapear.

© Healthicine

However, single illness elements are rare. Why? Single illness elements are often easily, even unconsciously, cured by natural healthy actions. Illnesses become more noticeable and more difficult to cure when illness elements combine to create composite illnesses, which require multiple cure actions. Diagnosis is a judgement. Many conditions are not severe enough to be diagnosed as a disease until a compound illness is present, until it has advanced to the point where multiple cures are required. This can create an illusion that the disease is incurable.

Composite illnesses have more causes – persisting even when one cause is addressed, when one illness element is cured. There are two basic types of composite illnesses; compound illnesses and complex illnesses, which can be combined to create compound-complex illnesses and which, over time, create chronic illnesses. Just as compound interest generates more income over time, compound and compound illnesses can generate more illnesses over time, becoming more complex and more severe as causes grow and damage accumulates.

Compound Illness

A compound illness consists of two or more illness elements, diagnosed as a single illness or disease. It has two or more independent present causes and causal chains, one for each illness element.

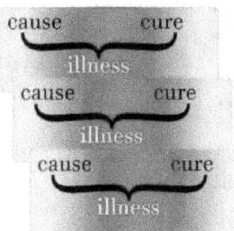

A Compound Illness

A **compound illness** consists of two or more illness elements having similar or overlapping negative signs and symptoms. It has two or more **present causes** which have often arrived at different times.

Compound illnesses are partially cured when any single cause is addressed, completely cured when all causes have been addressed and the signs and symptoms from those causes have faded and gone.

© Healthicine

Curing a compound illness requires addressing each cause with an independent cure. Sometimes what was seen as a compound illness element is cured with a single action. It has been resolved into a single illness element by the presence of a single cure. Cures prove cause.

Causal chain analysis might bring forth alternative solutions, or complications. Sometimes a causal chain splits in two, such that two independent causes each create the next link in the chain. At this point, our view of the illness changes from an elementary illness, with a single cause, to a compound illness with multiple causes. When a cause in the single chain portion is successfully addressed, a cure will result. However, addressing a cause at any point where two chains exist only produces a partial cure.

Secondary Illness

A secondary illness is an illness caused by an illness.

A Secondary Illness

A **secondary illness** is an illness caused by an illness.

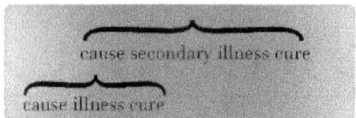

The causing illness might disappear while the secondary illness remains, or they might both be present, as a complex illness.

When the primary illness is gone, the secondary illness is usually an injury or an attribute illness, to be cured by healing or other transformation.

© Healthicine

A causal illness often causes another illness. Diabetes uncured causes many other illnesses. A causal illness might continue to cause more injuries, even as they heal, until the causal illness is cured.

An injury illness might cause us to change our habits and routines, perhaps resulting in changes to diet, exercise, or rest of body, mind, spirit or community, leading sometimes to health, sometimes to further injuries, or even to another illness.

An attribute cause persists until it is transformed and can have ongoing effects on many life activities, causing multiple illnesses.

Complex Illnesses

A complex illness consists of a present illness, the primary illness, and a secondary illness caused by the primary illness. Both illnesses are present at the same time. Thus, a complex illness consists of two or more present elements of illness with a single causal chain. The causal chain is extended by the chain of illnesses.

A Complex Illness

A **complex illness** consists of a present illness which is causing other illnesses. It requires at least two cures, one for the primary illness and another for each illness caused by that illness.

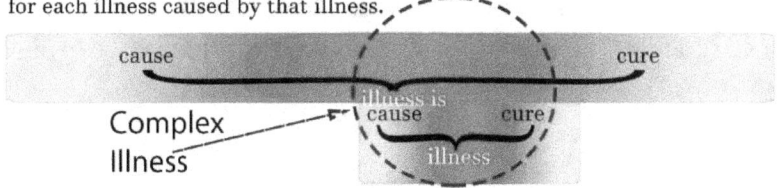

Treatments for the **secondary illnness** only address signs and symptoms. A cure must address the primary illness, the cause, or the secondary illness will to reoccur.

© Healthicine

There are 12 theoretical variations of complex illnesses: causal illness, injury illness and attribute illness, each creating a causal illness, injury illness or attribute illness. There are a few common types:

Causal Injury Illnesses – have a present process cause in diet, body, mind, spirit, community or environment, creating a single illness element which also causes injuries. These are probably the most common composite illnesses. When causal illnesses advance to the point where they cause injuries, they become *causal injury illnesses*. Two cures are required, a causal cure and one or more healing cures. In our current conventional medical paradigm, many causal illnesses are not diagnosed as a disease until injuries can be observed.

Attribute Injury Illnesses – consist of a negative physical, mental, spirit, or community illness attribute, which causes not just negative signs and symptoms, but also injuries.

Causal Injury Attribute Illnesses – have an active cause or a causal chain which is causing injuries that cannot be healed, creating negative attributes. Three cures are required, addressing the cause, a healing of the injuries, and a transformation of the negative attributes. A prolonged or severe case of scurvy can cause not just signs and symptoms – a causal illness, but also physical damage - injury illnesses, and also negative attributes which cannot be healed, can only be cured by transformations, and even permanent disabilities, from a single causal chain.

Complex illnesses require a cure for each illness element. Sometimes a causal cure allows injuries to heal, resulting in a cure of two illness elements from a single cure action.

Repeating Illnesses

Conventional medicine has little concept of repeating illnesses, and often refers to them as chronic.

An illness might be a single case, a set of repeating illnesses, or a chronic illness. The distinction is based on the cause. When the cause arrives, causes illness and then disappears and later recurs, the illness is repeating.

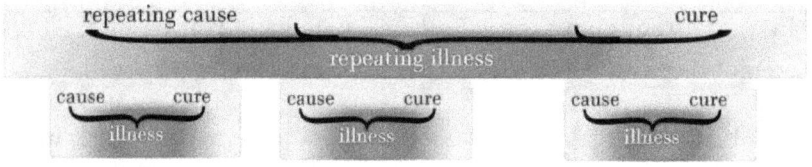

Repeating Illnesses

A **repeating illness** has a **cause** that *repeats*, creating **new cases** of illness until the repeating nature of the cause disappears or is addressed. Each individual illness is a new case **cured** by addresing individual instances of the cause.

The cure for a **repeating illness** is to address the repeating nature of the cause, a higher level attribute than the individual causes in each case.

© Healthicine

A repeating infection illness might occur when a person working in a kitchen has poor knife skills, resulting in many minor cuts, creating repeated infections. Repeatedly treating an infection having a process cause with an antibiotic, aiming to cure the infection-attribute, fails to see the repeating nature of the cause and fails to cure.

Repeating illnesses, like all illness elements and also chronic illnesses, can have causes in diet, body, mind, spirit, community, or environment, and cause signs and symptoms in body, mind, spirit, and community.

Repeating Diseases

There is an important distinction between a repeating element of illness, which has a repeating cause, and a repeating disease. Diseases can be diagnosed without reference to cause. As a result, it is possible for a new illness, with a different cause, to be identified as recurrence or extension of the *same disease*. If it has a different cause, it is a different illness, requiring a different cure.

Illness Duration

The duration of an illness is tied directly to the causes and recovery time after the cause is addressed. An illness cause might be of relatively short duration, like the common cold, or long duration, like prostate cancer, which takes considerable time to develop to a level of severity such that a diagnosis and cure is warranted.

Remember that an illness, by definition, can be cured. If it cannot be cured, duration is not relevant. A disability might last until the patient dies. When an illness can be cured, the duration is *until the illness is cured.* The current judgement of many incurable diseases is powerful evidence of our current inattention to cure.

When two or more causes are present, a compound illness is present, and multiple cures are required. Compound illnesses are stronger and longer lasting because they require multiple cure actions. Even two colds, or two influenza infections occurring at once, can present more severe symptoms and take longer to cure. However, our current medical systems have little ability to, and little interest in recognizing the presence of two cases any illness occurring at once. Diagnosis produces a single disease name. Treatments that do not cure do not attend to cause.

Chronic Illness

The US National Center for Health (sic) Statistics says a **chronic disease** is one lasting more than three months. It's a bureaucratic definition avoiding the obvious. Defining *chronic* by duration is a failure to comprehend chronic.

A chronic illness is chronic because *the cause persists over time*. There are chronic causal illnesses, chronic injury illnesses, and chronic attribute illnesses. Attribute illnesses are naturally chronic because the cause exists until it is addressed. Chronic illnesses can be simple, complex, or compound.

All chronic illnesses are attribute illnesses, because the causes have a chronic attribute that defines the illness. Chronic is an attribute of cause, not illness. Chronic signs and symptoms are a consequence of a chronic cause.

A chronic illness cause is often minor but persistent. In many cases, the cause provides health benefits. Often it's not severe enough to cause an illness without many repeated occurrences. No one gets smoker's cough, or lung cancer, from smoking a single cigarette. These chronic diseases are a result of a low-level cause that persists over a long period of time.

Chronic illnesses can be viewed as meta-illnesses, having a meta-cause or causal chain that repeats over time. They can be compound illnesses, where each individual element is below a level of diagnosis as a disease.

Chronic Illness

All attribute illnesses are chronic, caused by something that presists until the attribute is transformed. **Chronic causal and injury illnesses** are chronic because the cause is chronic. They often have a **cause** that provides some health benefits, and doesn't create illness until it occurs many times. The **illness** grows steadily until the chronic attribute of the cause is addresssed.

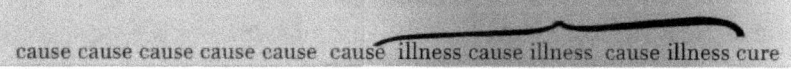

cause cause cause cause cause cause illness cause illness cause illness cure

All chronic illnesses are attribute illnesses. Addressing a single instance of the cause cannot cure. The chronic attribute of the **cause** must be addressed to **cure**.

© Healthicine

Any causal illness is chronic when the cause is chronic. The conventional medicinal definitions of three months, or a year in other cases, is an artificial distinction, ignorant of the cause of *chronic*. When the first element of illness occurs, there is no chronic illness except for attribute illnesses.

Chronic illnesses have longer durations because their causes persist over time, waxing and waning as the activities of the patient change, as healing waxes and wanes, often taking years to reach a diagnosable level. Even when the cause is not growing, the signs and symptoms and the damage can accumulate, growing more serious as time passes. Sometimes health and healing can compensate for a chronic cause for a long time – the illness only becoming noticeable as the individual weakens.

Smoker's cough might only appear after years of smoking, when a person's health begins to decrease noticeably. It rises and falls throughout the days, weeks, months and years. The cure might be obvious to doctor and patient, but the illness persists because of the complexity of the chain of causes, and the benefits provided by some elements in the chain.

Does the patient wish to continue smoking, with its physical, mental, spirit, and community benefits, or to cure their chronic cough, gingivitis, and prevent other diseases?

> *"Physician, heal thyself"*
> *Luke 4:23*

What doctor can cure themselves, and prove the cure? The only doctor who can cure smoker's cough is the doctor with smoker's cough. But there is no proof of smoker's cough cured.

Chronic illnesses are of short duration when the chronic cause is caught early. Other non-chronic illnesses might have a longer duration when the damage is severe, or the cure takes more time. Some chronic illnesses, like cataracts, persist until the damage is severe enough to warrant a dangerous treatment.

Chronic illnesses like obesity, or smoker's cough, can be caused by minor unhealthinesses that, in themselves, do not create illness. Over time, the effects of the chronic cause accumulate, and a chronic illness emerges.

Many chronic illnesses persist because the cause provides some benefits to the patient's body, mind, spirit, or community. Sometimes hard decisions must be made about curing or not curing.

> *"Wanting and not wanting the same thing at the same time is so common that we might even consider it a baseline condition of human consciousness."*
> *--- The Power of Not Knowing – Jamie Holmes*

A chronic illness might be due to an elementary illness with a single cause, persisting or repeating over time, or it might be a result of a compound illness with multiple recurring causes. Chronic illnesses can also emerge when a curable illness is treated for symptoms, with no attention to cause, with no intention to cure.

An infection might be a one-time occurrence, due to a single exposure to a dangerous bacterium. A chronic infection can occur when a person lives or works in an unsanitary environment.

A deficiency illness, like Vitamin C deficiency, might be a one-time occurrence when a sailor gets a temporary job on a ship with poor quality food, or it might be a chronic illness, caused by poverty, alcoholism, or ignorance having a chronic effect on the diet.

An injury illness can be chronic when the patient is chronically exposed to the cause. There are many common chronic injury illnesses, often called work-related injuries or repetitive stress injuries.

An attribute chronic illness might not be activated until a patient attempts a specific action – and is not judged an illness until that occurs.

Chronic illnesses accumulate when not cured. A patient with a chronic illness might acquire another chronic illness, and another, as conventional medical treatments treat signs and symptoms, failing to cure. A chronic illness can also cause a chronic illness.

When a person has repeating exposure to a cause, or to causes creating similar signs and symptoms, the disease paradigm sees a single disease. When a chronic cause exists, a simple cure becomes impossible. As a result, the disease paradigm views chronic diseases as incurable. Cured is not scientifically defined any chronic disease, even when a cure is trivial.

Chronic Pain

A common example of a chronic illness that can cause other chronic illnesses is the medical condition often called *back pain*. Back pain is a dog's breakfast of illnesses, with many potential causes. Each unique cause has many potential cures. There are dozens of books claiming to cure back pain, each with their individual theories and stories of success. Most view back pain as an attribute illness, cured by some physical transformation, sometimes by a causal process. Conventional medicine treats back pain as an injury illness, with medicines to mask signs and symptoms and waits for healing to cure. Successes are seldom called cures, even when a cure occurs. Cures of chronic diseases are ignored by the conventional medical system. The phrase *placebo effect* is often used to rationalize ignoring success that comes from a non-medical treatment.

It is possible, of course, for a person suffering back pain to have two causes, or more, accumulated over time, to be in need of two or more cures. Our medical system often aims or settles for measurable relief from symptoms, euphemistically defined as *works*. With back pain, it can be difficult to distinguish between a massage that provides relief from pain and a massage that transforms a physical blockage, curing an illness. When cured is not defined, when cure is not the goal, there is no interest in the distinction between a treatment that cures and one that *works*. A distinction that can become more difficult when multiple back pain illnesses are present.

Curing gives relief because it is a cure, not because it is an effective treatment for every patient with back pain. However, today's medical systems make no such distinction. Back pain cured is not defined.

As a result, back pain becomes chronic. Few doctors attempt to cure it. Those who succeed are ignored. There are no cases of back pain cured in conventional medicine references – cured is not defined. Even when our back pain is cured, we might fall into a permanent cure trap, believing the illness might go away and come back later. This is simply a misunderstanding about illness. An illness is not something that can go away, or hide, and return. When the cause is addressed or goes away naturally, it is cured. When the cause returns or reoccurs, it creates a new illness.

Degenerative Diseases

Degenerative diseases are chronic conditions that cause more and more damage over time. The damage might result in injuries, negative attributes, or disabilities. Degenerative diseases have chronic causes, chronic causal chains that exist, repeat, and persist over time. The cause might be a process or attribute that the patient can change, or it might be an attribute, feature, or a disability, which the patient cannot change themselves. Some cases are incurable conditions, some are curable illnesses.

Type 1 Diabetes is believed to be a degenerative disease, due to a disability – the absence of islet cells. Type 2 Diabetes, on the other hand, is viewed as a degenerative disease believed to be caused by the patient's life choices. As a result, Type 1 Diabetes is viewed as an incurable degenerative disease, not a curable illness. Type 2 Diabetes is a potentially curable degenerative illness. However, today's medical practice does not have any technique to recognize a case of diabetes cured when it occurs.

It is important to emphasize *viewed as.* Type 1 Diabetes and Type 2 Diabetes are complex and varied illnesses. It might be possible for one patient to have an incurable Type 1 Diabetes, a disability, while another patient has a curable Type 1 Diabetes, a curable illness. We cannot know for certain until we succeed in curing. It is also possible for one patient to have an incurable Type 2 Diabetes illness, while another has a curable Type 2 Diabetes illness. We only know for certain when we cure the illness.

If a case of diabetes is incurable, it's a disability, not a curable illness. It can, however, be a cause of illness. Judgements of incurable need to be challenged for cures to be attained, even for a cure to be recognized.

There are many complex and compound illnesses, with causes leading to signs and symptoms, that become causes leading to more signs and symptoms. We can only break chains of illness-caused illness with cures.

Beneficial Diseases

We rarely think of diseases as being beneficial. Sometimes an illness prevents or cures another illness. Sometimes illnesses improve overall healthiness – after our natural healthiness cures them. These concepts are seldom explored in a medical system bent on selling products to treat signs and symptoms of disease with few attempts to cure.

Many have suggested that influenza is a healthing disease. The concept is simple, like a forest fire that enables new growth. As our body, and our cells become less and less healthy over time, we become susceptible to many diseases. The flu virus attacks and kills the weaker cells- and then burns out due to lack of fuel. The weaker cells are replaced by new, healthier growth. After the flu the patient is healthier than before. Conventional medicine has little interest in this theory – and no tools to study it scientifically.

Measles is another interesting case. We have recently learned that a case of measles can cause the immune system to forget what it has learned. Could measles be a cure for some autoimmune diseases? In our eagerness to eradicate measles, or to promote the measles vaccine, we ignore this possible cure.

Diseases are not simple. Many diseases are beneficial sometimes, some can cure other illnesses. However, because we rarely recognize cured, we can recognize cured by disease either.

Idiopathic Illnesses

In today's medical paradigm, many conditions are judged to be idiopathic. Idiopathic is defined as *"arising spontaneously or from an obscure or unknown cause"* (Webster's). There are no *spontaneous* illnesses. Every illness has a cause. The phrase idiopathic illness, in the practice of medicine, is often an excuse to treat signs and symptoms, and avoid further investigation of cause.

Incurable?

At present, cured is not defined for most diseases. Cured is not defined for any non-infectious disease, from arthritis and Alzheimer's to bloat, Chron's, cancer, depression, diabetes, gout, hypertension, obesity and even scurvy. Without a definition of cured, we might consider them all incurable in *the absence of theory*.

A medical condition judged to be incurable might be a disease, disability, a handicap, or a natural feature. When a decision, or diagnosis, or medical practice judges a condition to be incurable and it is subsequently cured or is later judged to be curable, it has been transformed by the presence of a cure, into a curable illness, but only if a cure can be recognized.

A causal condition judged to be incurable might be a disease, but not a curable illness. A patient with Type 1 Diabetes, judged to be incurable, has a disability, not a curable illness. If it can be cured, or if it is cured, it was converted from a disability to a curable illness. An injury judged to be incurable is not an illness. It has become a condition that must be accepted. A patient whose leg is blown off by an explosion has a disability, not a curable illness. Of course, until the injury is healed, they also have an injury illness. What appears to be negative attribute illness, when judged to be incurable, becomes a reality that must be accepted and dealt with, not an illness to be cured. Cataracts were judged to be a disability until we learned to cure them with surgery. Specific cases might still be judged an incurable disability.

Too Depressed, or Two Depressed

Is depression an illness, or several illnesses? Is it a simple illness, a complex illness, or a compound illness? Is it a repeating illness, or a chronic illness? Might it be a single illness element in one case, and a serious chronic illness in another case? Is it possible to have two depression illnesses at once? Is it a degenerative illness? Is depression a curable illness or an incurable disability? Sometimes? All the time? Illnesses don't have names without a diagnosis. In our current medical paradigm, it might be a disease, or a symptom, or medical condition – the distinctions are seldom clear.

Dr. Kelly Brogan has written a book about depression, **A Mind of Your Own**, in which she views depression as a symptom, not a disease.

Symptoms cannot be cured, and many diseases can't be cured either. Only an illness element can be cured – by addressing a causal element.

Depression, as defined in the Diagnostic and Statistical Manual of Mental Disorders, is a *symptom domain.* The DSM does not use the word disease. It appears that, according to the DSM, a simple depression illness with a single present cause, is not diagnosable. Our health cures it naturally, with minimal effort in a relatively short time. If a case of depression can be cured by health, there is no need for treatment, so it's not a diagnosable disorder. The difference between a curable depression and an incurable depression? An incurable depression can be diagnosed. A physician can use the DSM guidelines to diagnose a patient's depression and prescribe a medicine to treat (*not cure*) the depression. There is no diagnostic test for depression cured. The DSM advises doctors on how to diagnose mental conditions, but not how to treat mental conditions, not how to cure, not how to recognize cured. There are no statistics for cures of depression. Officially, no one is cured. Depression is technically an incurable disorder, due to the absence of a definition of cured.

Clinical studies of depression measure signs and symptoms and effects of treatments. They do not define cured, so cures cannot be detected, much less documented. A recent search of ClinicalTrials.Gov for the keywords *depression* found over 6400 clinical trials, but when restricted to having the word *cure* there were only found 29 references. Not a single study defined cured. Most references to cure were variations of incurable. Some refer to treatments, without a cure goal, as *cures,* others to *hope for cure*. Depression is incurable in conventional medical practice, by lack of a definition of cured.

Dr. Kelly Brogan tired of treating depression disorders with medicines. She decided to learn to cure depression illnesses. Brogan doesn't use the term illness, but her definition of a symptom is close to the healthicine definition of an illness. The concept of a causal illness, as the intersection of a cause and consequences, does not exist in conventional medicine, so Dr. Brogan is stuck between words like disorder, or disease, and symptom – although none fits the situation and none points to a cure.

Dr. Brogan treats depression as a causal illness. She treats depression by finding the present cause of the symptoms and addressing that cause. Sometimes, she treats the depression as an injury illness, to be cured by rest and healing. Sometimes she treats it as an attribute illness, to be cured by transforming negative attributes of the patient. Sometimes she treats a causal illness, identifying causal processes in the patient's life. Sometimes, all three types of cures are needed. The cure in each case is health. Dr. Brogan cures depression by improving healthinesses. She identifies causes of depression as absences of healthiness and healths depression.

A Mind of Your Own has many stories of depression illnesses cured. Every cure is a single patient, who has an illness, with a causal chain, often multiple causal chains. The illness is cured by addressing the causes. Every cure is an anecdote, a story. Some patients have compound and complex depression illnesses. Some cases are long and complicated requiring multiple cure elements.

It is possible to be depressed, to be suffering from a single illness of depression. It is also possible to be more depressed, to be suffering from a more severe depression illness. It is also possible to be suffering from two (or more) independent depression illnesses.

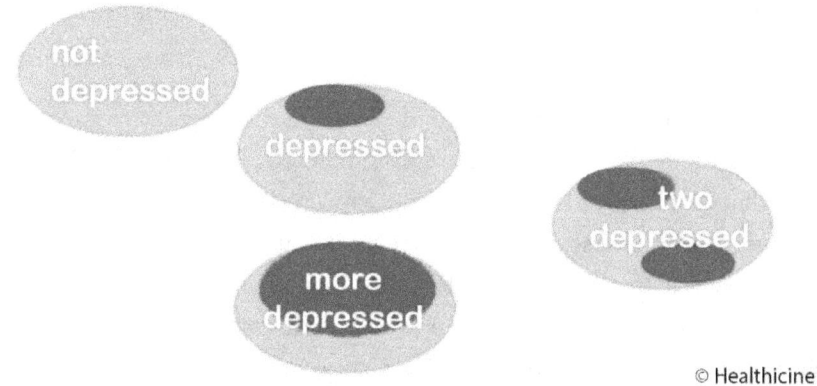

This image shows the differences. A patient is two depressed when they have two causes of depression, requiring two cure actions. It is possible for a patient to have many causes of depression – each of which must be addressed for the disease to be cured.

Most, perhaps all, of the patients that Dr. Brogan treats have a compound depression illness, with two or more active causes; two or more depression illness elements. Some have complex depression illnesses, with depression causing depression, requiring time-consuming complex cures. People with only a single depression illness are often cured in a short time – by natural healthiness. Depression is more likely to be diagnosed as a disease only after it becomes a compound illness, when it is harder to cure. Curing a single element of a compound illness leaves the patient *still depressed,* and the result can be... depressing. The patient and doctor might easily give up, easily reactivate the cause that was addressed, acquiring the cured illness element again, moving back to the status of having two depression illnesses, without doctor or patient recognizing the causes.

We know how to make someone depressed. Depression illness has many causes, and we can control most of them. Depression can be caused by loneliness, lack of community support, recent stressful life experiences, marital or relationship problems, trauma or abuse, financial strain, alcohol or drug abuse, dietary deficiencies, dietary excesses, unemployment or underemployment, other health problems, chronic pain, and more. We can easily give someone depression. We can easily give someone *two depression illnesses* at once. We can intentionally make their depression more and more by making the causes stronger and more and more compound by adding causes.

Let's pick one: dietary deficiencies. If someone is suffering from a specific dietary deficiency, they will become depressed. Some dietary deficiencies don't cause depression, many cause minor depression, and others can cause severe depression. A minor deficiency of amino acids can cause a minor depression. A more severe deficiency of a specific amino acid can cause a more severe depression. A deficiency of an amino acid doesn't cause *two depressions.* How do we know? Because there is a single cure.

A recent stressful experience, the loss of your job, the loss of a parent, the loss of a child, can cause depression. In medical-speak, in medical diagnosis, it's the same disorder: depression. From a cure perspective, they're different illnesses. They have different present causes, similar symptoms, the same diagnosis, but different cures.

One and one make two. If you are suffering from a deficiency of amino acids, and then you suffer the loss of your job, you might suffer two depression illness elements, one physical based, and one spirit based. When we consider the possible causes of depression, it's easy to imagine someone to be suffering from three, four or more depression illnesses, requiring multiple actions to cure.

Our medical systems treat depression as a symptom. When they only treat depression symptoms, it's easy to believe a patient with three depressions is *more depressed,* to prescribe a *stronger medicine.* However, often, the person is not depressed more, they have more depression illnesses – an important distinction. It gets worse. Severe depression is depressing. Medicines used to treat depression can cause side effects that are depressing. Chronic depression can also cause changes in the brain which might require a transformation to cure. Causal depression can lead to an attribute depression illness, when not cured.

Kelly Brogan cures depression. She rarely uses the word cure. It's forbidden for doctors to claim cures.

Depression is cured with health, not with medicines. Dr. Brogan cures depression with health. She cures by addressing the causes, by healthing her patients. When a cause of depression is successfully addressed, a single illness element has been cured. It might appear that nothing was cured or that the depression disease is only less severe.

One cause has been addressed; one illness cured.

Many of Dr. Brogan's depression cures take a long time. One of the cures she presents is Eva, who took a year to cure. Eva was on several medications, treating multiple depressions. She was also taking medicines to treat symptoms caused by medicines to treat symptoms of depression, none of which made any claim to cure. It's no surprise it took so long to address that depressing accumulation of causes.

Dr. Brogan does not use a term like *multiple depression illnesses,* although she treats multiple depressions, by addressing multiple causes. When a patient has multiple depression illness elements, the compound depression disease won't be cured until each of the chronic causes is addressed, until each of the illness elements is cured. When we view compound depression as multiple illnesses, in the same patient at the same time, we can understand more about each case, and how to cure it.

This also prompts us to think differently about other diseases named depression by our medical systems. Is manic-depression one illness? Or could it be two illnesses, each fighting for control? Or maybe sometimes it's one illness, and sometimes it's two illnesses. The only way to understand a specific case is to address its causes, to cure each illness element. Sometimes we might identify a cause by accident, addressing it without understanding, and then observe the result. We might think it was just placebo effect. A placebo cure is a result of addressing a cause we are not aware of, a cause we don't understand.

Treatments with drugs offers little hope of a cure. They seldom address causes. Sometimes drugs might appear to *help a patient with signs and symptoms* until time when their body, mind, spirits and communities find a cure in health. A drug might help the patient get through the time required to cure – but we must aim to cure.

It is also important to understand that depression can be a sign of healthiness. Sometimes illness is like a weed. A weed is only a weed when it is judged to be a weed. In other cases, it might be a beautiful flower or a useful plant. If you are depressed because of loneliness, and you take a drug to help with signs and symptoms your depression, you might be making yourself less healthy, pushing the depression symptoms down, without any effort to address the cause. A social activity like volunteering might address the cause, provide purpose – improve spirit healthiness – and cure the illness.

Curing depression can be hard and time-consuming, and it can be difficult to tell if you are cured. Cured is when we believe the cause has been addressed, when we believe a cure is present because the cause has been addressed.

Dr. Brogan cures depression; she gives us hope that every case of depression is curable. We can only cure depression, as we cure any illness by making the patient healthier, by addressing the causes of each depression illness element.

Is it possible that some cases of depression are disabilities, or handicaps, and therefore incurable? We don't know. Perhaps some depression illnesses are caused by negative attributes and can only be cured by difficult transformations.

We can only know when we work to cure every case of depression, and then give up on some. A disability exists when we give up trying to cure.

Signs and Symptoms

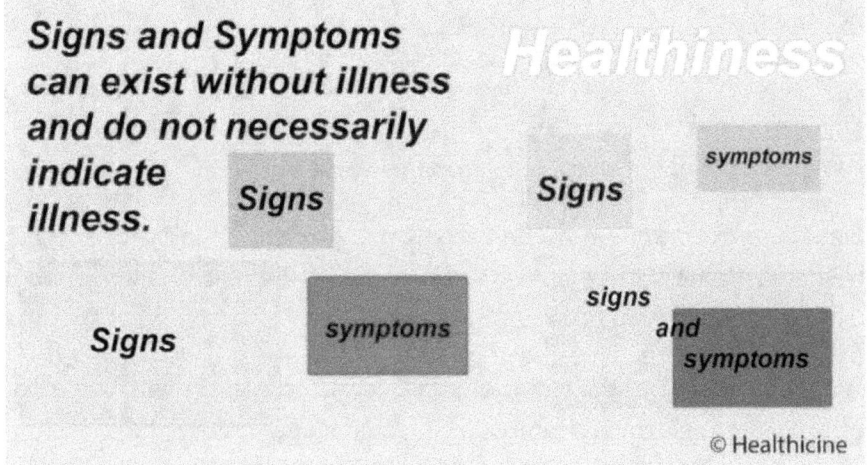

It is important to remember that there are signs and symptoms of healthiness, as well as signs and symptoms of illness. *I feel great!* is a sign, a symptom. Spring fever is a symptom of vitality, of health.

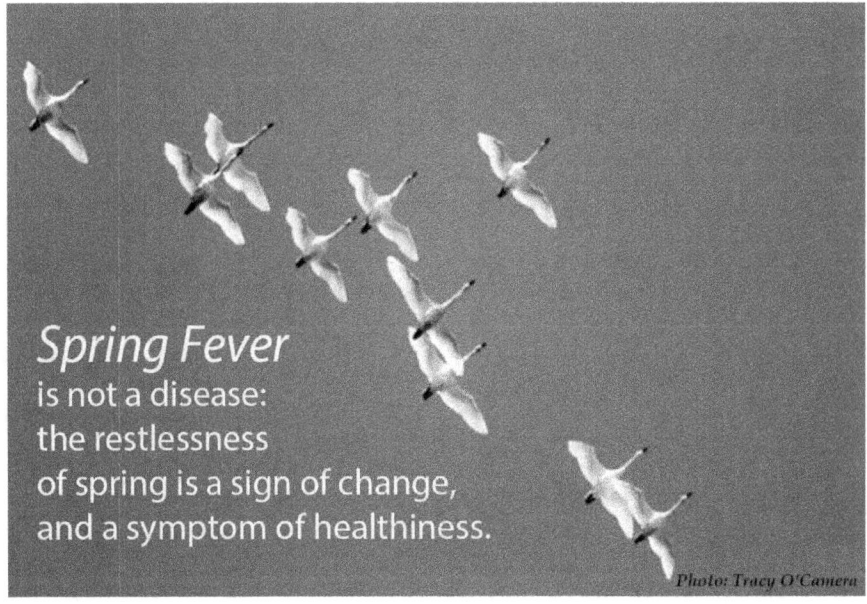

Signs and symptoms of illnesses are usually, but not always, negative consequences of the illness. Every sign, every symptom of an illness provides information about the illness. In addition, it can be difficult to determine if specific signs and symptoms indicate illness or natural healthiness.

Signs and symptoms cannot be cured. An illness can be cured. When illness is cured, signs and symptoms fade away. Some damage is healed, some damage might become a permanent feature.

Signs and symptoms not addressed by a cure might indicate another element of illness to be cured, a non-illness, a disability, handicap, or a natural feature which does not need curing.

We might itch from the touch of an insect, from contact with a poison, or from healing, which prompts us to scratch and remove the cause and promote healing. A specific itch might be judged healthy or unhealthy.

We might cough because of a cold, an illness, or we might cough because water went down the windpipe – a healthy cough.

We might experience or observe many signs and symptoms we cannot connect to a cause. We are often uncertain which signs and symptoms are linked to an individual cause. We might only prove a link by curing the illness, and, even then, never be perfectly certain. When the illness is cured, does certainty matter? Masking signs and symptoms is a deliberate action to hide some aspects of the illness, helpful for many short-term illnesses. Often harmful with chronic illnesses, often assuming incurability, seldom moving any illness towards cured.

Side Effects

Side effects are unintended negative effects, signs and symptoms, of treatments and cures. Treatments can have positive and negative effects on a patient's health and on various aspects of illness. Side effects are often iatrogenic signs and symptoms, sometimes iatrogenic illnesses – caused by medicines or treatments that decrease healthiness, often with no cure goal.

Cures can also have side effects. Every action to improve healthiness consists of give and take. The negative effects of a cure are, like every illness and every cure, judgements. A cure for our cold or influenza means we can no longer pamper ourselves in bed watching television. Many people with illnesses, especially chronic illnesses, become attached to their disease, or some aspect of it, and consciously or unconsciously don't want it to be cured.

> *Paradoxically, we make ourselves ill*
> *in order to take care of ourselves the best we can.*
> *--- John Harrison, M.D.*
> *Love Your Disease: It's Keeping You Healthy*

Causal cures sometimes decrease enjoyment. Healing cures often have side effects while the curing process is active – congestion, itchiness, or pain. Cures by transformation can have many side effects because they entail significant changes to diet, body, mind, spirits, or communities. Curing can be difficult. Insignificant changes being less likely to cure.

Congestion

Congestion is often a consequence, of injury and illness. It can also cause injuries and illnesses.

Congestion can occur when a natural flow is blocked, or when an unnatural or unhealthy flow cannot be released or cleared. Sometimes internal leakages cause internal congestion. Our nasal passages get congested when we have a cold. Our minds become congested when our spirits are depressed, blocking healthy activities. Our streets are congested when everyone tries to go to work, or the lake, at the same time, creating unhealthy traffic flows.

Congestion can sometimes arrive suddenly. It often grows slowly, almost imperceptibly, progressing as we grow older, accumulating and building in force. Congestion might remain hidden for long periods, being cleared by natural, healthy processes, until a person attempts an action that blocks a healthy flow, or until a process flows faster than it can be cleared.

The cause might be internal or external. Many internal body parts are external to other parts. Many simple illnesses cause temporary blockages or leakages, leading to temporary congestion which is naturally cleared by healthy activities and healing.

Congestion can be cleared, but if the cause is not addressed, the underlying illness will not be cured, and the congestion will reoccur.

Today's medical practice, in general, is to treat symptoms. Congestion is often viewed only as a symptom of illness, treated with a decongestant. Sometimes an illness is short-term – like the common cold – and a decongestant is effective and appropriate. At other times, treating congestion, while ignoring the cause, can allow illness to persist, grow, and perhaps to multiply. Like all signs and symptoms, congestion speaks to us, provides valuable information about the underlying illness. When we suppress symptoms, we can fail to understand, and thus fail to cure.

No medical professional would advise a patient to *"learn to live with their congestion"* while many might advise a patient to *"learn to live with their hypertension."* High blood pressure is a symptom of illness; a congestion, due to unhealthiness in the blood vessels, that might be cured with health, but not with medicines.

Congestion might also be a result of a disability, a handicap, or a natural attribute which cannot be cured. We may need to continually clear congestion from a disability because we cannot cure the disability. The congestion will be a chronic symptom, recurring as long as the patient lives. In these cases, the congestion is a sign and symptom of a disability, not of illness.

Elements of Cure

*Everything should be made as simple as possible,
but not simpler.*
Albert Einstein

Cure: (noun). A cure is the end of an illness. An action that brings about the end of an illness. After a cure, medicines are no longer needed.

'A complete or permanent solution or remedy.' Merriam-Webster's College Dictionary 11th Edition, 2003, 3.

Cure: (verb). To bring about the end of an illness in an individual life entity,

"To bring about a recovery from disease." Merriam-Webster's College Dictionary 11th Edition, 2003

Three Elements of Cure

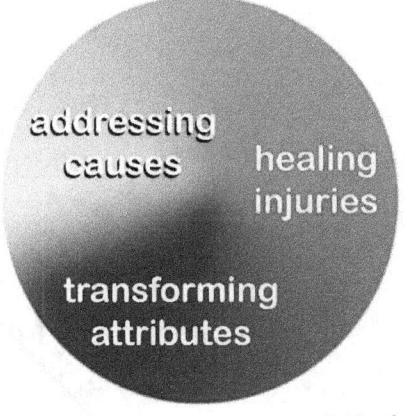

© Healthicine

There are three elements of cure, based on the three elements of illness, which are based on three types of cause.

Each cure addresses a present cause. Past causes cannot be addressed. Potential causes are speculative and do not cure any illnesses.

Causal process illnesses are cured by actions that break the causal chain, addressing the active causal process.

Injury illnesses are cured by healing the present injury to body, mind, spirit, or community. Healing progresses naturally regardless of cause, and may be aided or hindered, by physical, nutritional, mental, emotional, spirit, community, or other factors.

Attribute illnesses are cured by transforming present negative attributes into neutral or healthy ones. The action of transforming might cause injuries which need to be healed.

Types of Cures

The three basic processes are curing, healing, and transforming. Cures must address the present cause. Preventative actions and clearing congestions are often viewed as cures, but rarely cure.

An elementary cure addresses the single cause of an illness element. Each elementary cure is simple in principle.

Each type of illness element has a unique type of cause, and thus requires a unique type of cure, as this chart illustrates.

cause	>> illness	>> cure
Unhealthy Process	Causal	Address Cause
Severe Stress	Injury	Heal Damage
Negative Attribute	Attribute	Transform Attribute

© Healthicine

Curing: (a causal cure) brings about the end of an illness by addressing the causal chain of faulty process of diet, body, mind, spirit, or community.

Healing: (a healing cure) – ends a present injury by healing the damage. Healing is seldom perfect, those who expect perfect cures will find few.

Transforming: (a transformational cure) addresses a negative attribute of diet, body, mind, spirit, community or environment. Surgical cures are transformations, but most transformations are much less severe. Exercise of body, mind, spirit, or community can bring about a transformational cure, causing permanent or lasting physical, mental, spirit or community changes.

Compound Cure: a set of cures for a compound illness, an illness with multiple independent causes.

Complex Cure: a set of cures for a complex illness, an illness with a single cause and multiple illness elements.

Meta Cure: an action that cures a chronic illness or cures several illnesses or diseases at once. A healthy diet might be a meta cure that addresses scurvy, beriberi, and other nutritional deficiency illnesses all at one time. When an illness causes another illness, a cure for the first illness might cure both. When we cure illnesses with health, meta cures sometimes occur.

Chronic Cure: cures a chronic illness by addressing the chronic attribute of the cause. Sometimes, the cause persists at a lesser severity or frequency without causing illness, after the chronic attribute is addressed. Chronic cures often require a transformation of some present, or current aspect of the patient, their habits or routines.

Natural Cure: a cure from nature, as opposed to intentional curative actions. Any illness might be naturally cured over time. Our lives change as time passes. Our bodies, minds, spirits, and communities change. Our habits and routines change. When a life process changes, even without intention, sometimes without awareness, an illness might be cured. Injuries are healed naturally, by natural healing processes. An attribute cause of illness, like a scar that interferes with movement, might fade over time and the illness fades as well.

Life is naturally healthy, naturally curative. Health cures a common cold, the flu and measles – even as no medicine can cure. Healing is a natural cure. Time does not *heal all wounds.* It facilitates healing of injuries and natural transformations of negative attributes. Causal illnesses might be cured by natural activities or events that address the cause without conscious intention. A single action, unintentional or unintentional, might cure a complex illness by addressing the cause, while natural healing cures injuries. Chronic cures, like all cures, sometimes come naturally from health, from natural, healthy activities which address a cause and its chronic attribute without intention. Every cure has a cause. There are no spontaneous cures.

SAD is an illustrative example. Seasonal Affective Disorder is a temporary chronic disorder, cured naturally by the passing of time, of the season. It might be argued the illness is still present and will return next winter. No. Next winter, the cause returns and causes a new case. However, if the patient moves to the tropics, the illness might never be caused again. The argument that it was not cured because the cause will make it recur is simply a misunderstanding of cured. Every illness can occur again if the cause comes again. Illnesses are not things. They cannot go away and return. Causes can disappear and later reoccur, creating a new illness.

There exists much fatalism in the medical view of cures, such that *if the illness might return* it was not cured. This view is simplistic and not useful to define cure, nor to find cures. Every illness cured by addressing a present cause might occur again when the cause arrives again, or if a similar cause arrives. If the cause has been successfully addressed, the illness has been cured. A new arrival of cause is a new case of illness.

There is no difference between a sailor who gets a deficiency because of the poor food on board a ship the first time, and a second time, years later from a similar or completely different cause. Each case is a new illness, with a new cause, the second is not a *recurrence*. Inability to understand the link between causes, illnesses, and cures often creates this confusion. We might say that the sailor *"should know,"* but that's a different judgement, not related to the distinction between a new illness and a recurrence. Remission is a remission of signs and symptoms, not of cause. Signs and symptoms might fade and return, due to healing or other natural processes. Illnesses are present or absent when causes are present or absent.

Cure Variations

Cured is a positive judgement. Of course, judgements can be wrong, but to cure, we must judge cured. There exists a decision point, a judgement, where the cause and consequences are judged to have been addressed. At that point, the illness is cured. Cured has many variations.

The common cold is cured when the patient's health addresses and overcomes the cause, when the signs and symptoms have faded and gone, and no more medicines are necessary. Another cold might arrive, sooner or later. A new cold does not nullify the cure. The cure was complete - not partial, final - not temporary.

Similarly, a patient with an illness caused by a poison might be cured when the source and poison are removed. A new case of poisoning, not a remission, occurs when a similar cause occurs again. Injuries caused by the poison might be able to be healed, or permanent disabilities.

Chronic illnesses are especially difficult for conventional medicine to judge as cured, for two reasons. First, causes of chronic disease are chronic, not simple. Second, due to the nature of a chronic cause – only chronic attribute illnesses can be cured by a medicinal treatment. Chronic causal or injury illnesses can only be cured by changes to the patient's life processes, habits, and routines.

Cures for chronic illnesses, and for illnesses caused by excesses, often seem like miracles, because the illness has already lasted a long time, and because no medicine or single action caused the cure. All cures might appear to be miracles, until we understand the cause of the illness, until we understand the cause of the cure.

Complete Cure – all elements of an illness or disease are cured. Depending on the damage done by the illness, a complete cure might require life changes, healing, and transformation. The cause and injuries, and any resulting attribute illnesses of a complex illness need to be addressed. The patient no longer suffers the effects of the illness and no longer requires medication. A complete cure is seldom, if ever, perfect. Each cure element addresses a single element of illness. Together they can completely cure a complex or compound illness. A complete cure cures an illness, not a patient.

We often think of a cure as a magical event, where all traces of the illness are gone, and healthiness is totally restored. Magical cures are not realistic. We often need to accept some permanent consequences of illness, even as we cure.

We can adapt the Serenity Prayer to understand cures better: *"give me the strength to cure illnesses that can be cured, the serenity to accept those that cannot be cured, and the wisdom to know the difference."* If it cannot be cured, it might be a disease, but not a curable illness. Every curable illness has the potential to be cured, but not every consequence of illness.

Partial Cure – a partial cure can occur when the present cause of a causal, injury, or attribute illness is partially addressed, and the patient experiences relief from effects of the illness. The need for medication might be reduced. Relief from signs and symptoms does not necessarily indicate a partial cure. It is possible to relieve signs and symptoms even as the illness worsens. Addressing signs and symptoms is only a cure, when their presence is causing a secondary illness.

Partial cures are common:

- when a cause in the causal chain of an illness element is only partially addressed
- with a complex or compound illness a partial cure exists when some, but not all illness elements are cured.
- when an injury is partially healed
- when a negative attribute is partially transformed

Complex and compound illnesses often need to be cured one partial cure at a time. It can be difficult to recognize a partial cure because some illness is still present. Conventional medicine has no concept of partial cure at present.

Temporary Cures exist when the cause of an illness is temporarily addressed. It can be difficult to distinguish between a temporarily cured illness and a chronic or repeating illness. Temporary cures might lead to chronic illness. Temporary cures although common, are also not recognized, and often denied, in current medical practice.

A weight loss diet, for example, can be a temporary cure, whereas a permanent change in diet can be a permanent cure. Dieting can lead to chronic illness, seldom to cures. Dietary changes might lead to healthiness and cures, other chronic illnesses, or both in some cases.

Medical publications tend to view cures as temporary and questionable for most diseases. These are failures to understand cures and the concept that an illness is cured when the cause has been addressed. Failures to believe in cures creates failures to cure.

Maintenance Cures Causal illnesses can only be cured by creating or changing habits or routines to address a cause, which must be maintained to maintain the cure. A healthy diet cures Vitamin C deficiency, but the healthy diet must be maintained to maintain the cure. Sometimes an exercise cure transforms the patient, resulting in an attribute cure, a permanent cure. But when the cause is an absence of exercise, an exercise cure is a maintenance cure, only persisting as long as the patient persists in the exercise. When the cause is an excess of exercise, like shin splints, the cause must be maintained to maintain the cure. However, some cases of shin splints might be cured by improving healthiness and healing, converting the illness into a cured injury.

Illness Can Cure Illness Sometimes an illness cures another illness. Perhaps this sounds counter-intuitive? There are many ways for it to happen. Many illnesses are a result of a severe imbalance or inability to balance – in body, mind, spirit, or community. Sometimes a new illness moves the balances in the opposite direction, curing an illness. Many illnesses cause transformations – and sometimes an illness causes a transformation that cures a different illness. A sailor might develop a Vitamin C deficiency while working on a ship that provides an unhealthy diet. If the sailor gets sick with a different illness, they might be dropped off in a port, where their diet changes to a Vitamin C healthy diet. We might say that the second illness cured the deficiency illness. Of course, if the sailor goes back to work on the ship, they will get a new case of Vitamin C deficiency.

Remission is the absence, or diminishing of signs and symptoms, with the continued presence of the cause. Many medical references confuse remission, where the signs and symptoms of illness are diminished, with cure, where the illness is gone. Why? In today's conventional medicine, cured is seldom defined and cannot be validated. Claims of remission do not need to be validated. There is no medical test, no scientific test, no definition of remission of a disease, only for remission of signs and symptoms.

Remission can be brought about medically by treatments designed to address signs and symptoms, but not cause. Remission is not a cure, no matter how long it lasts, although many cures can be mistaken for remission. Remissions might be followed by further decreases in healthiness, even to chronic illness when the cause is not addressed.

Distinguishing between remission of symptoms and cure is easy in theory. A cure exists when the present cause has been addressed. There is a gradation between having the cause addressed and having the cause still present. Many illness causes, once addressed from the perspective of causing illness, are still present, but no longer causing illness.

Health is Whole

Health is whole. The word health is based on the word whole. Historically, health refers to wholeness, completeness, and soundness. It is important to understand that a body that is seen to be incomplete in some way is still *a whole body*. No individual is perfectly healthy, perfectly sound, but each is a whole.

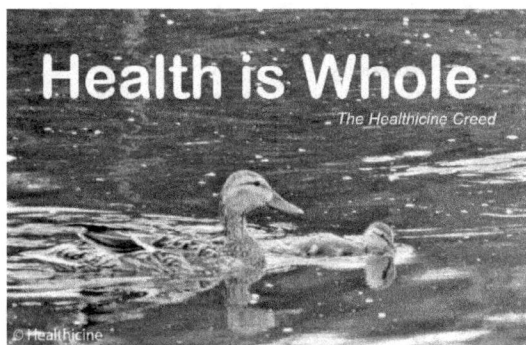

An individual's healthiness includes their whole body, their whole mind, their whole spirit as well as the wholeness of relationships and interactions with their communities.

Health is always whole. When we measure any individual aspect of healthiness, we are measuring a wholeness that consists of its healthiness and its unhealthiness, which together sum to 100 percent.

The health of a baby duck is whole. The health of an adult duck is also whole.

The health of an aged senior is whole. A younger person might be stronger, without being healthier. It is not possible to be *more whole.*

The health of a disabled person, someone missing an arm, or a leg, is a whole. When we look closely, we might see that everyone is disabled in some ways. Everyone's health is also whole.

The psychopath might appear to be two people, of two minds, but in truth, we are all of two minds, more or less at some time in our lives. We each have many spirits, many intentions and life goals, sometimes in conflict with ourselves. It's healthy to do so. Perfect health is not possible. No-one is perfectly healthy, we each have room to improve our healthiness.

> *Perfect health, like perfect beauty, is a rare thing; and so, it seems, is perfect disease.*
> *-- Peter Latham*

The goal of life, the goal of health, is to live, to move forward in time. Perfection is perfectly stable. Perfection is dead.

The wholeness of health includes the potential for improvement. Someone who is in perfect health is someone who has no unhealthiness, no room for improvement. They can only make choices, only take actions that decrease healthiness. Perfection in health cannot be attained and if attained in any dimension, cannot persist if the individual is to live.

Healthiness and Unhealthiness

Health is whole, consisting of healthiness and unhealthiness. We can view the combination of healthiness and unhealthiness as the yin and yang of health.

When a healthiness grows in one direction, towards the yin, it moves the inverse, the yang, in a different direction, towards the yang. We eat healthy foods to be healthy, but too much food is unhealthy. We need healthy exercise of body, mind, spirit, and community. Too much, or too little, becomes unhealthy.

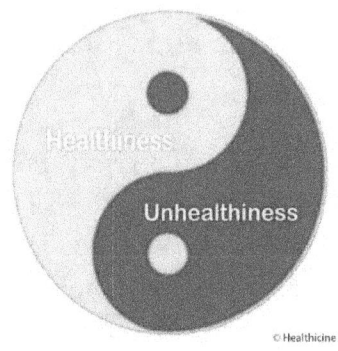

A healthiness is a specific measure of healthiness and unhealthiness. Each yin and yang of health, every healthiness, contains the seed of the corresponding unhealthiness. Every unhealthiness contains the seed of its corresponding healthiness. Health is about life, not about perfection. Each healthiness must compete, must actively balance with others for life to progress. Good health comes from balancing of yin and yang, which allows other balances to function, to balance and imbalance, to maintain life.

Health is whole. We can only measure healthiness on a percentage scale. Healthiness and unhealthiness are inverses of each other. As healthiness rises, unhealthiness shrinks. As unhealthiness climbs higher, healthiness shrinks. Health is whole; thus, any individual measure of healthiness also contains an opposite measure, of unhealthiness.

Together, a specific healthiness and its corresponding unhealthiness add up to a whole, to 100 percent.

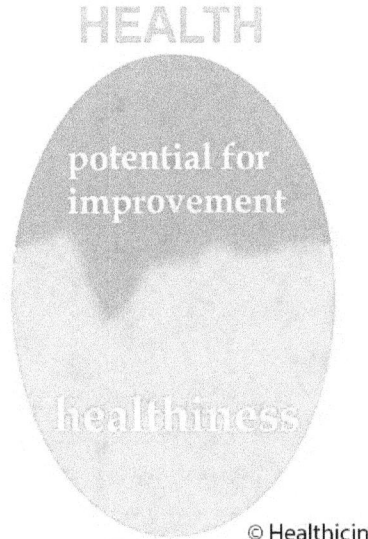

There is another important way to view unhealthiness. We can view unhealthiness as *potential for improvement* in healthiness, as in this diagram.

If something cannot be changed, cannot be improved, it is a reality that must be accepted, dealt with, sometimes used to advantage. But it is not an unhealthiness. Healthiness and unhealthiness are factors which can be changed.

Over our lifetimes, our healthinesses fluctuate up and down, a natural, healthy process. A person might have 80 percent weekly exercise healthiness with 20 percent unhealthiness over one period of their life and a score of 60 and 40 percent over another period.

An individual healthiness is measured as a ratio or a process over a period of time and compared to a goal – 100 percent healthiness. The goal is required to produce a percentage score. Different time periods give different views of healthiness. Life exists over time, not in the moment. Specifying the period is often an important aspect of measuring healthiness. Longer or shorter periods of measurement result in different answers. Measurements over short time periods often measure only signs and symptoms, less effective in measuring healthiness.

Examples of healthiness can include things like:

- consumption of a specific nutrient or necessity of life over days, weeks, months.
- amount of time asleep, awake or drowsy, over a day or week.

A healthiness can be specific, as above, or more general:

- weekly exercise routine
- average daily consumption of some nutrients, weekly consumption of others
- weekly, monthly, or seasonal variety in diet consumed
- daily consumption of common toxins like alcohol or caffeine
- habits and routines

The definition of a healthiness might be very specific, the daily consumption of an individual nutrient, or very general – summarizing many measures of healthiness together to create measures of healthiness of body, of mind, of spirit, of the entire person, even their communities.

Healthinesses are constantly moving up and down the scales of healthiness and unhealthiness.

Health is Whole: Healthiness and Unhealthiness are the opposing components of the whole

100 — Zero
Percentage of Healthiness
Percentage of Unhealthiness
Zero — 100

As healthiness rises, unhealthiness shrinks
As healthiness falls, unhealthiness grows

© Healthicine

Each measure of healthiness is a measure of status and potential. Measuring potential is hard. *"If you think you can, or you think you cannot, you are right."* It's a useful mantra. Sometimes it is impossible to achieve what we believe possible, and sometimes we succeed to our astonishment – when we believed only failure could result.

Healthiness: Body, Mind, Spirit, Community

Each aspect of healthiness has a physical component in the body, the diet, and the environment, a mental component in the mind, an intention component in the spirits, and a community component which joins our individuality with our communities. These components are supportive. When we are less healthy in body, our mind, spirit, or community might compensate. When we think we can, we can. When our friends or our communities think we can, we can.

It can go the other way. When our community is unhealthy, it can create unhealthiness in body, mind, and spirits. When are our spirits are unhealthy, we fail to look after ourselves and our communities. When our mind is unhealthy, the bad decisions we make affect body, mind, spirit, and community.

Illness: A Hole in Healthiness

All illness comes from an absence or deficiency of healthiness.

This statement seems obvious, trivial. It is a useful view, not a perfect view. We can use it to study and understand cures. A healthiness is a specific aspect of health.

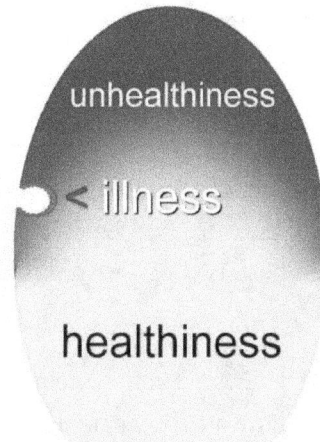

An illness is a hole in health

Illnesses can appear when unhealthiness grows too large, when healthiness shrinks, or from external causes

Health is still whole.

© Healthicine

An illness is a hole in a healthiness that occurs when healthiness falls so low there is a damage or disruption to body, mind, or spirits or community.

Healthiness to Illness

Over time, each aspect of healthiness rises and falls naturally, some more than others. Usually, they don't fall far enough to cause illness, as in this next diagram.

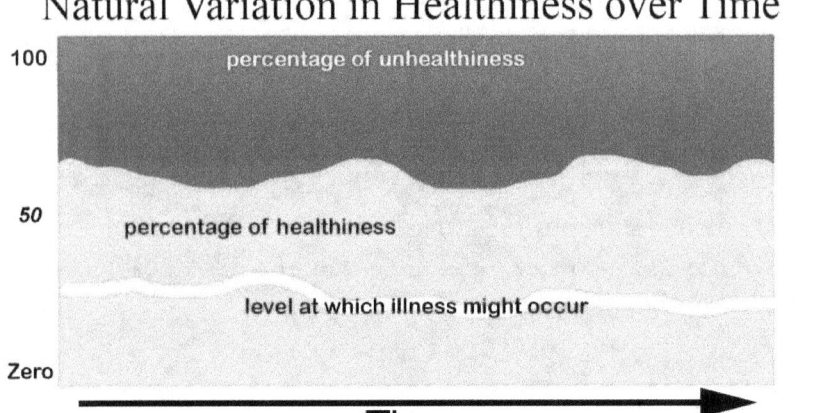

When healthiness falls, unhealthiness grows, and illness might be occur.

A causal illness is a failure in the processes of life, resulting in a severe absence of healthiness, a hole in healthiness. There are two basic types of causal illnesses: deficiencies and excesses. These two causes result in different progressions of illness.

When designating an illness as caused by a deficiency or a stress, we must distinguish between past and present causes. Many attributes, including most injuries, are caused by stresses in the past. We might prevent future illnesses by addressing these causes, but to cure a present illness, we must address the present cause.

Deficiency Illnesses

Deficiency illnesses are always in waiting. When healthiness drops too low, illness emerges. A deficiency illness is cured directly by raising healthiness. Healing and passage of signs and symptoms might take time.

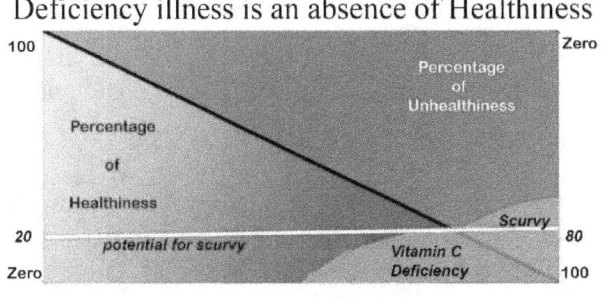

Vitamin C deficiency and scurvy illnesses occur when healthiness drops so low that a hole occurs.

Most deficiency illnesses are causal illnesses. Deficiency illnesses are holes in healthiness that emerge when healthiness drops too low due to a deficiency of a specific necessary of health.

The potential for Vitamin C deficiency and scurvy is always present. We might say scurvy occurs when Vitamin C healthiness falls below X percent. While Vitamin C healthiness is maintained above X percent, there is no scurvy. Scurvy can only be diagnosed when the Vitamin C deficiency becomes severe – which takes time. Over time, the deficiency becomes more severe. We can use a similar model for any deficiency illness, an illness caused by lack of iron, or exercise, or sleep. Simple deficiencies result in illnesses consistently when the deficiency is present. More complex healthinesses, like loneliness, can be countered by other aspects of health and might not cause illness until severe or long-lasting. Some illnesses can raise the need, raise the need of other healthinesses necessary to prevent illness.

Sometimes a deficiency occurs because needs rise. The current medical model of recommended consumption of Vitamin C ignores the fact that sometimes we need more Vitamin C to meet specific life stresses. In animals that can manufacture their own Vitamin C, this can be handled naturally, but in humans, it must be addressed by consumption.

Some illnesses, like bedsores, are caused by a deficiency of stress. Deficiency of stress is also a stress. Boredom might be caused by a deficiency of physical, mental, spirit, or community stress, which can then lead to illness. We need healthy levels of stress to be healthy. Illnesses caused by a deficiency of stress might be cured by healthy exercise of body, mind, spirit, or community, even if the initial deficiency is not directly addressed. Once we get moving everything moves.

Conventional medicine today has no concept of unhealthiness and no standards for measuring healthiness. Numbers indicating the presence of illness based on cause are rarely standardized.

Before and after a cure, the potential to cause a deficiency illness is always present. Perhaps this is the reason many references avoid the word cure with regards to deficiency illnesses. This is a simple misunderstanding of the concepts of illness, cause, and cure. A deficiency is not something that can go away and return. It is the *present absence* of something necessary to health.

A deficiency cause of illness might a deficiency of process, stress, or an attribute of diet, body, mind, spirit, or community. All three types of illness can be caused by a deficiency. A deficiency of process, like a dietary process, leads to a causal illness, cured by a process. A deficiency of stress can lead to an injury illness, like bedsores. Injuries are cured by healing, but the illness will continue, grow, or recur if the deficiency is not addressed. The deficiency of an attribute can be, or lead to an attribute illness, which is cured by a transformation. We sometimes determine what type of illness was present by observing the cure.

Illnesses Caused by Excess

Illness can occur when healthiness falls, or when stress rises. The stress might be internal or external. Stress might be caused by a deficiency. But perhaps we shouldn't call a deficiency a stress illness, to avoid cure confusion, because we identify the illness as caused by a deficiency, or by a stress, to guide cure actions.

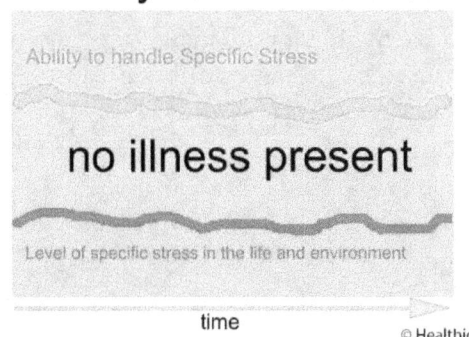

Healthy Level of Stress

Life forms use stress to get things done. We need to tolerate stress even to manipulate and make use of stresses in life. The cause and effect processes of life cannot function without forces, without stresses.

Bacteria are always a present and healthy part of our environment. Normally, healthiness is maintained above the level where a bacterial infection occurs. Sometimes, they can multiply to illness causing numbers, regardless of the level of healthiness. When healthiness falls, when unhealthiness grows, infectious bacteria can take advantage and create an infection.

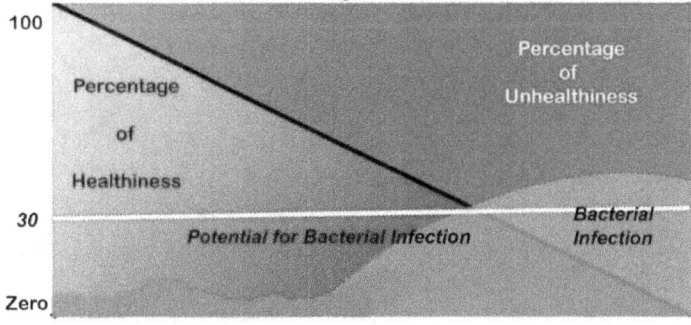

Stress illness Emerges from Unhealthiness

Development of illnesses caused by stresses is more complex than deficiency illnesses. A bacterial infection does not emerge automatically when a healthiness falls. A fall of healthiness presents an opportunity for bacteria. Our bodies, our skin, our healing and immune systems, and healthy activities like washing provide additional protection. Healthiness protects against illness.

Stress illnesses can be caused by excess stress from diet, body, mind, spirit, or community. Stress illnesses might be causal illnesses, caused by an ongoing stress that results from natural living activities. Stress often causes injury illnesses – and we might view all injuries as caused by stress of some time. Stresses caused by negative attributes cause attribute illness.

Judgements and Closure

"You cannot see the wind, you can only see that there is wind." G.K. Chesterton

Health is whole. An illness is a hole in health, like a hole in a donut. We can see the hole in a donut. When we eat the donut, it disappears. Was it really there?

When we cure an illness, by addressing the cause, the illness disappears. Was it really there? We cannot see an illness. We cannot touch an illness. We might see the cause. We see or feel the consequences, the signs and symptoms. We sometimes refer to the signs and symptoms as the illness, but this error leads us away from cures. A non-injury illness is not a thing; it is an invisible intersection of cause and consequences.

An illness is a concept, invisible. When we treat symptoms, it's like covering the hole of a donut. The hole in a donut is not part of the donut. It is part of the *not donut*. When we cover the symptoms of an illness, we might make them disappear, but the illness is still there. We just can't see it. We never did see it.

Mom: *"You're sick. I'm going to take your temperature."*

Son: *"I'm fine mom, just a bit tired."*

When does something rise to the level of an illness? How can we be certain an illness is present?

An illness is a negative health condition with a cause. Negative is a judgement. Every health condition, positive or negative, is a judgement.

When is an illness judged to be present? A disease is judged to be present at diagnosis, but an illness is usually required exist before a disease can be diagnosed. Many disease diagnoses do not require a curable illness to be present. An incurable disability or handicap can be diagnosed without a reference to a curable cause.

Illness is a Judgement

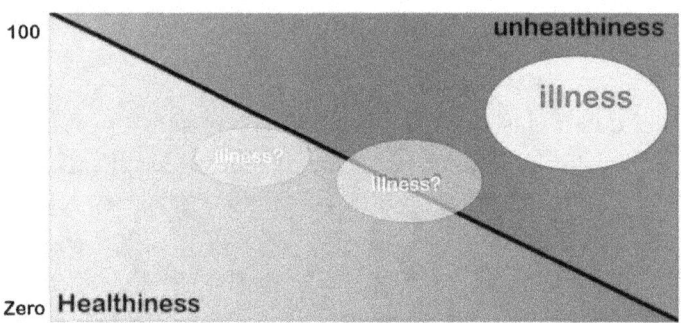

As healthiness drops, when does illness appear?

© Healthicine

As healthiness falls, illness appears as a hole in healthiness. When does an illness exist? How big a hole is necessary?

One person might perceive an illness and another not. A doctor, or a friend, might notice an illness the patient ignores or denies. A patient might fuss or fret over an illness that is denied by the doctor.

We use many different words to describe sickness, illness, disease, medical condition, which we might expect to be cured, and also for negative conditions we do not expect to change. *"He's sick,"* or *"he's ill,"* might mean he has an illness, like a common cold, or *"he is sick,"* that he enjoys hurting people, that he is a sadist. We don't expect a cure. Maybe we should?

A curable illness is a negative condition in a life entity; an intersection of cause and negative consequences, which we believe can be cured. Every illness is a negative judgement. The presence of an illness depends on the judgement of the patient or the doctor. We might compare some illnesses to a mass of dandelions. To a young child or a grandmother, a field of yellow blooms might be viewed as a delight, an opportunity to make tea, or wine. To a landscaper or a golf course manager, they are a blight, needing to be killed. An illness might distress a patient, and be dismissed by a doctor, or be diagnosed by a doctor and dismissed by the patient. It's complicated. Of course, many illnesses, like weeds, are almost always viewed in the negative. But, for example, a case of mental insanity might be judged differently depending on the viewpoint and goals of the prisoner, doctor, lawyer, or the court, and each viewpoint might change over time.

A case of disease is different from an illness. It is still a judgement. The diagnosis of a disease is a judgement by a medical professional. Disease is defined more clearly – although many diseases are defined without reference to cause. Definitions of diseases are designed to be general, while each case is unique, having unique features. A case of disease only exists after a diagnosis – which might be current, or retroactive, and might be right or wrong. Different doctors can often produce different diagnoses or the same patient. *"The incidence of diagnostic error in medicine"* by Mark L Graber, published in BMJ Journals in 2013, suggests that *"the diagnosis is wrong 10–15% of the time."* When a diagnosis is not available or is incorrect, an illness might still exist.

There are no easy answers. Medical researchers and theorists work to simplify disease diagnoses, to make them more certain. But the more we work to clearly define each disease – especially if diseases are defined without reference to cause, the more spaces appear for errors and for illnesses to fall between the definitional cracks. This is important because diseases are often defined without identifying a present cause and the causal chain which might be different in different cases.

Cause: A Judgement

We often view cause and effect of illness as facts, like scientific facts. No cause is a fact in itself. Every cause has a cause. We can deconstruct any cause into a set of many lesser causes. Which cause is important to cure? The present cause, that when addressed, produces a cure.

> Mom: *"You didn't wear your sweater last night, now you're sick."*
>
> Son: *"It's not that, mom, I think I was just up too late. I'm tired."*

Every cause is a judgement. We are never certain something was the cause of a cured illness, nor the cause of a cure in a specific case. We can only exercise our best judgement. Conventional medical techniques of diagnosis prefer signs of illness, which can be seen and measured independently, and validated by other people. This has strengths and weaknesses. It is independent of the patient – a positive and a negative. It is highly dependent on external information, which might be relevant or not.

Clinical studies base causal judgement on statistics, which provide stronger general knowledge, while blurring and missing information from individual cases. Every illness is an individual case. Every cure is an individual case.

The signs and symptoms of an illness can affect the diet, body, mind, spirits, and community of the patient. When we notice signs and symptoms, it's natural to look for a cause, to look for preventatives, to look for a cure. Causes surround us. Be aware: many causes of illness can also be causes of healthiness.

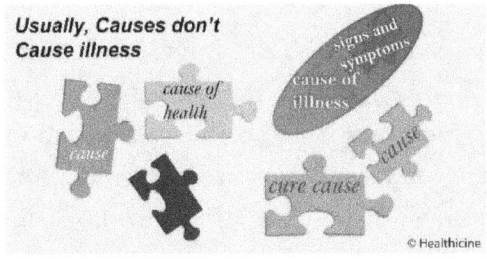

Cause and effect come not from illness, not from healthiness or unhealthiness; but from life. Life searches causes and effects, and uses them, for the health of it.

Causes of cures also surround us. Every cure has a cause. Every successful cure action is the cause of a cure.

Most things we identify as causes do not cause illness most of the time. We can consume healthy amounts of many nutritional substances, to support our health. Illness can occur with consumption of excessive amounts or when consumption is deficient. Causal illnesses have causes that are actions or processes, not things. Healthy actions foster healthiness; unhealthy actions can lead to illness, but a judgement of healthy or unhealthy depends on the individual situation.

Cured: A Judgement

Mom: *"I see you're better now. That cold medicine worked."*

Son: *"It took like a week mom. I don't think it helped at all."*

How can we know for certain that an illness has been cured? How can we know if the treatment action caused the cure?

Every cure is also a judgement. We know that a diagnosis is a judgement. We trust our doctor's judgement or seek a second opinion. According to current published research, many doctors refuse to make a judgement of cured. We should not be surprised. Cured is seldom medically defined. Doctors are not trained to diagnose cured. Conventional medicine has no techniques. There is no training to diagnose cured for most medical conditions, much less to determine the cause of a cure.

The cause of an illness element might exist in the diet, body, mind, spirit, community, or environment of a life entity. We explore causes in the past, the present, and the future. However, only present causes lead to cures. The consequences, the signs and symptoms of illness can affect the diet, body, mind, spirits, communities, even the environment of a life entity.

The cure of an illness might come from an external source, by addressing the cause, by making the patient healthier, or from the natural health of the patient.

Incurable: A Judgement

> Son: *"You'll never cure that cat of jumping up on the table."*

Can an illness be incurable? Yes, and no. Incurable is also a judgement made in a specific case which cannot be proven. It is impossible to prove that any case of a disease or an illness is incurable, we can only decide to accept a disability, handicap, or other attribute that cannot be cured. Any claim of incurable might be falsified by a cure.

> *Science is built on falsification, not proof.*
> *When you lose that insight, the humility of the genuine*
> *skeptic is replaced by the arrogance of scientism.*
> Robert J Frey on Twitter

When a condition is judged incurable, it is no longer a curable illness. Judging an illness incurable converts it to something else, perhaps a disability, a handicap, or perhaps a natural, positive or negative feature or attribute of the life entity.

When we claim an illness is curable – the claim cannot be falsified. We might give up attempting to cure it, but that does not prove it incurable.

Thus, Barron's Dictionary of Medical Terms defines incurable as *"being such that a cure is impossible **within the realm of known medical practice.**"* Incurable conditions are made curable by a cure.

Closure

Jamie Holmes, writing in Nonsense: The Power of Not Knowing speaks to our natural need for closure in judgements. Our need for closure affects our judgements about illness, about causes, about cures, and about incurables.

> *Need for Closure: Desire for a definite answer on some topic, any answer as opposed to confusion or ambiguity.*
> *--- Arie Kruglanski*

Our need for closure naturally varies over time and according to the situation. When we are stressed by an illness, for example, our need to know rises, and we are grateful for a doctor who gives our illness a disease name, even if they declare it incurable. When we are suffering, we don't want to hear that every diagnosis is a judgment, that every cause is suspect, that incurable is a judgement, that every case of cured is a judgement.

Doctors need closure as well, and get primary closure through diagnosis. Diagnostic closure is important, but premature closure leads to mistakes. Patients want closure, and doctors often aim to deliver closure in the face of ambiguity. In their practice, doctors often need to consciously lower the need for closure. Lisa Sanders, in Every Patient Tells a Story, writes, *"By far the most common diagnostic error in medicine is premature closure – when the physician stops seeking a diagnosis after finding one that explains all or most of the key findings, without asking... what else could this be?"*

Diagnosis provides a certain level of closure, that might be validated or raised to a higher level by further analysis. A cure is the highest level of closure possible for an illness.

We might think that closure is critical in the theory and practice of medicine, but actually, the right level of closure is critical.

The need for action and closure is directly related to urgency. Injuries often have high urgency, and therefore a high need for action, which requires closure.

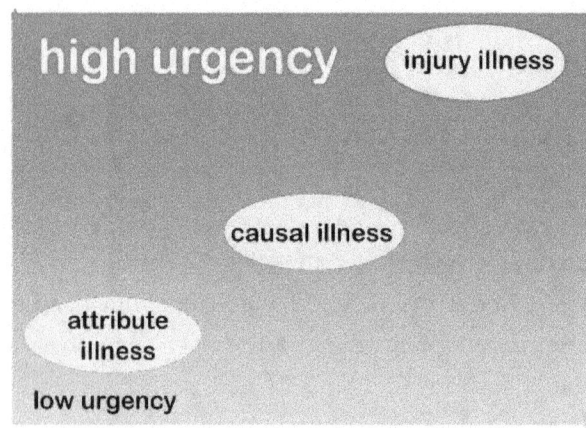

As urgency rises, need for action rises raising the need for closure

© Healthicine

Chronic illnesses and attribute illnesses often have low urgency, and low need for closure, until they cause severe injuries.

There is a high need for closure in emergencies. When any illness creates an emergency, decisions must be made, and delay can be dangerous, might even kill.

On the other hand, when a patient has a low-level chronic illness, closure that does not cure is of little importance. A diagnosis provides sufficient closure for a treatment recommendation. However, diagnosis of a chronic disease seldom provides a cure, often providing a false sense of closure.

A cure provides the most complete closure. Causal illnesses which have not yet caused injuries have a medium need for closure. When not cured, they can cause injuries with a higher need for closure. Unfortunately, many causal illnesses cannot be diagnosed as diseases until injuries occur.

The cure of any illness element is an anecdote, a story. Stories need closure. As an illness becomes more complex, closure becomes more elusive. In novels, individual chapters have less closure. The goal is to maintain the story, not to close. History books don't provide closure, by design.

We can relate this to illness, by comparing single cures, to multiple cures, to clinical studies of treatments, to meta-studies of disease. As we move from specific cases to general cases, the level of closure falls.

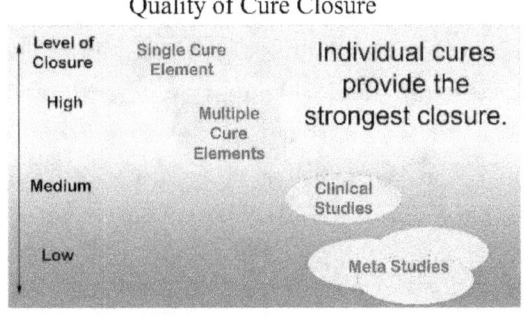

We might, mistakenly, think that knowledge and closure are stronger or higher with clinical studies and meta-studies. The reverse is true.

Most clinical studies and meta-studies do not provide closure. They measure benefits of treatments that do not cure, that provide no closure in individual cases.

Cure closure is strong for individual illness elements, weaker when multiple illness elements need to be cured. Some elements might be easily cured, others more difficult. Cure closure is not present in clinical studies and meta-studies unless the study measures cures. Cured is currently not defined in most clinical studies, which place value on *results within study parameters*. Clinical studies seldom measure cures, and when they do, closure is lower due to the number of independent variables from each new patient, diagnosis, cause – or causal chain. Even clinical studies that cure seldom cure every patient. They are designed to test a specific treatment – no to find the right cure for each patient.

Meta-studies have extremely low cure closure. They intentionally avoid individual cases and rarely examine cures.

Current conventional medical thinking places more value on clinical studies and meta-studies than on individual cases. The high value placed on clinical studies and meta-studies is a consequence of judgements that seek closure for treatments, but not for illness, not for cures. The consequences are a predictable: a surplus of treatments that do not cure, and a dearth of cures.

When we have a high need for closure, Jamie writes *"we tend to revert to stereotypes, jump to conclusions, and deny contradictions."* Clinical studies measure diseases, as stereotypical illnesses, not as individual cases. Meta-studies are studies of stereotypical studies of stereotypes of diseases. Imagine what a meta-study of a cure would measure? It might measure the quality of the cure, not the quality of the treatment. As far as I am aware, there are no meta-studies of cures.

Drug marketers need treatment closure. They have little interest in cures of individual patients. The primary goal is profit. Drug marketers sometimes need to raise ambiguity (decreasing closure) for the competition, about *alternative treatments* (competitive treatments) while increasing our belief (raising closure) in their medicine. Maybe you've noticed, or maybe not, that drug advertisements sell anxiety more than cures. *"Talk to your doctor about...."* The goal is to close the sale, not to cure any patient. Anxiety sells drugs. The marketing mantra *"sell the sizzle, not the steak,"* is converted to *"sell the treatment, not the cure"* in medical marketing.

Identifying an illness is a judgment. Every judgement provides a specific level of closure. At the same time, every judgement is tentative. Identifying a cause of illness is a judgement. Each judgement moves us towards closure. Every cure is a judgement. Every cure provides closure, but judgments of cured are tentative. This is a reality of curing.

Every declaration of *incurable* is a judgement. Judgments of incurable are tentative, never providing closure.

How can we manage all this ambiguity, and still search for cures, and for cured?

We can act. We can make cures our goal and take actions to achieve those goals.

We begin with judgments. We must tolerate and work with ambiguity. Judging an illness as the intersection of a cause and a set of consequences is the first step to a cure.

Then we move to cause. If we want to cure an active illness, we must find a present cause to address. Every potential cause is a judgement. Once we make a judgement, we can test it. We can test causes. When we address a cause, it cures. Testing cause provides closure, the illness was cured, or not cured. Even a failure to cure by testing a potential cause provides valuable information – either that was not the cause, or our actions failed to address it.

Judging cured is essential to curing. Every cure is a judgement. Maybe it's not a real cure. Maybe it's just a change in signs and symptoms. Maybe it's just temporary. Maybe it's just a remission of signs and symptoms. Maybe it's a partial cure. When a cure first occurs, we have less certainty. We gain knowledge and certainty over time, but only by aiming to cure. When we aim to diminish signs and symptoms – we lose sight of valuable information, drift farther from cures. Only as we build success finding and understanding cures, can we improve our ability to cure.

Managing closure is an important factor in finding cures. When our need for closure is too high, it leads to errors. When it is too low, we don't care enough to seek cures. When we are ill, our need for closure can easily rise too high. We need to seek other opinions, to consult our communities and our doctors. Doctors need to provide balance in closure, in order to find cures.

> *Cure: to remove legal defects or correct legal errors.*
> *Black's Law Dictionary*

It's interesting that a law dictionary provides a clearer definition of cure than any medical text. The strongest forms of closure are found in our law courts. However, legal decisions are extremely specific, anecdotal. Each case is unique and must be decided based upon individual details. Legal decisions do not aim for general understanding; instead, they build general knowledge by answering very specific legal questions. At the same time, any legal decision might be tentative, subject to appeal.

A stronger legal decision, with stronger closure, often contains less general value. The more general value a closure decision provides – the less value it might bring to specific situations. And so it is, with cures. Stronger cure closure comes in individual cases, not in clinical studies.

Cures

Health is the best preventative. Health is the best cure.
- The Healthicine Creed

Health is the best cure. It is most effective to look for health first, to take a healthiness view of every illness, every cause, and every cure.

Medicine is a practice where each patient's illness is an individual case. Diseases provide the meta-view. When no disease can be diagnosed, conventional medicine is often at a loss for treatment recommendations. Even when a diagnosis is available, medicine seldom looks for cures, instead, the standard of practice is to treat signs and symptoms. Most clinical studies measure success by measuring signs and symptoms – even to the point of ignoring cures. This is a powerful technique for incurable conditions, seldom effective for curing. Treating signs and symptoms *works* according to the parameters defined in clinical studies, even as it fails to cure.

Each element of an illness requires a single, unique cure element. Conventional medicine has no concept of an element of illness. Many, perhaps most diseases consist of multiple elements of illness requiring multiple cure elements. A cure, and the definition of cured depends on the specific illness element being cured. Lumping illness elements together into a disease lumps causes together, resulting in failure to cure, failure to see causes and cures of illness elements, even cures occur.

As mentioned earlier, many medical dictionaries and references do not contain the words cure, cures, curing, nor cured. Use of the word and the concept of cure is inconsistent. I have yet to see any medical definition that links a cure to a cause. Perhaps part of the reason is the difficulty proving cured. Most medicines cannot cure. The other reason I believe cure and cause are not linked is the confusion from analysis of past (and future) causes. Only a present cause leads to a cure.

Health, not medicine, is the best cure, often the only cure.

Cures: Bacterial Infection

The easiest, perhaps the only illness, that the practice of conventional medicine can cure and prove to be cured, is an infection. Let's begin our study before an infection occurs.

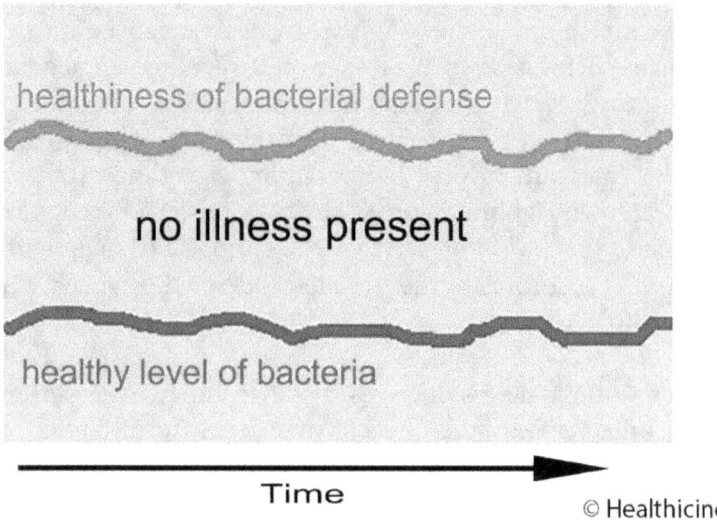

This diagram illustrates levels healthiness changing over time when there is no bacterial infection. Bacteria are always present in the environment, an essential part of healthiness. Without bacteria, all life on the planet would cease to exist.

There is a healthy gap between the person's bacterial defenses and the bacteria present. So long as the bacteria does not overwhelm the defenses, there is no illness.

Most dangerous parasites, like tapeworms, are rare in today's environments. A healthy environment is the first layer of a healthy defense. Health is the best preventative. Most bacteria are commonplace, even healthy, only causing illness when they multiply out of control.

Curing Bacterial Infection #1

In this diagram, we see bacteria overwhelming the patient's healthy defenses, causing an illness.

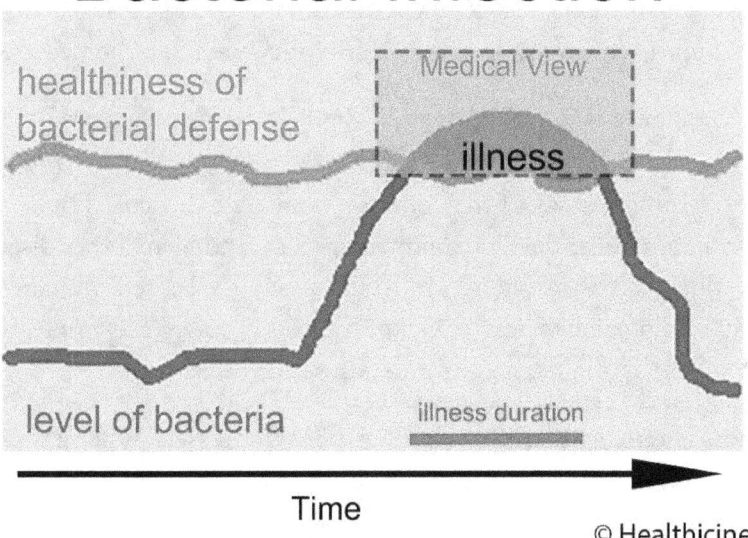

The red shaded box views an infection from a conventional medical perspective. It only represents a small part of the larger image. There is no treatment in this diagram. When a person has an infection, the health of the patient normally overwhelms the parasite, and the illness is cured naturally. Healthier patients cure infections faster, more effectively. I wonder how often conventional medical and alternative medical practitioners claim cures that are brought about by health. Of course, cure claims by alternative medical practitioners are often dismissed with *placebo effect* mysticism.

Most infections do not advance to the point where medicines are required. When bacterial infections are treated with antibiotics, the illness is perceived as caused by bacteria. However, many infections are cured with health. A dentist treating infected gums, for example, understands the recommendation *"treatment goals for gingivitis are to identify and eliminate the factors that are making the person more susceptible to gum disease."* These healthy actions cure – but such cures are not counted. Instead, the words used are *treatment* and *treatment success*.

If the patient's illness is advancing dangerously, or their health is unable to overcome an infection, a medical antibiotic cure might be necessary.

When the illness is cured by health, there is no test for cured. Thus, conventional medicine says, *"There is no cure for the common cold,"* even though most cases of the common cold are easily cured by health. The common cold, influenza, mumps, measles, and many other diseases are described as self-resolving. In truth, no illness is a self; no illness is a physical thing, much less a living entity. Illnesses are resolved by healthy cures, by healthy actions to address the cause.

An illness is cured when the cause has been addressed. Whether it was cured by health, or by a medicine, should not affect a cure judgement.

Curing Bacterial Infection #2

The following diagram illustrates another cause of a bacterial infection.

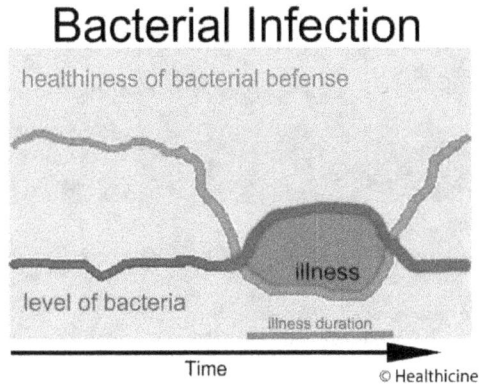

An infection can occur when the patient's defenses fall below the threshold necessary to hold back an overgrowth of naturally occurring bacteria.

This might happen due to an injury or an immune system deficiency.

Once bacteria overwhelm the weaker defense system, they can grow and create a serious illness. This is the gingivitis example from dentistry. In many cases, the infection is cured by health. Sometimes a medicine is used to fight this type of infection. However, using a medicine to kill the bacteria can be the wrong treatment, even if it succeeds. Medicines can *work* even as they fail to cure. Medicine produces a temporary cure and is easily perceived as a correct treatment. It does not address the cause, might even weakness in the patient's bacterial defenses allowing other illness to occur. The unhealthiness cause was never addressed – the illness was never cured. The medicine only put the signs and symptoms into remission, without addressing the cause.

Curing Bacterial Infection #3

In the first case, we viewed the illness as caused by the bacteria. In the second, as caused by poor health.

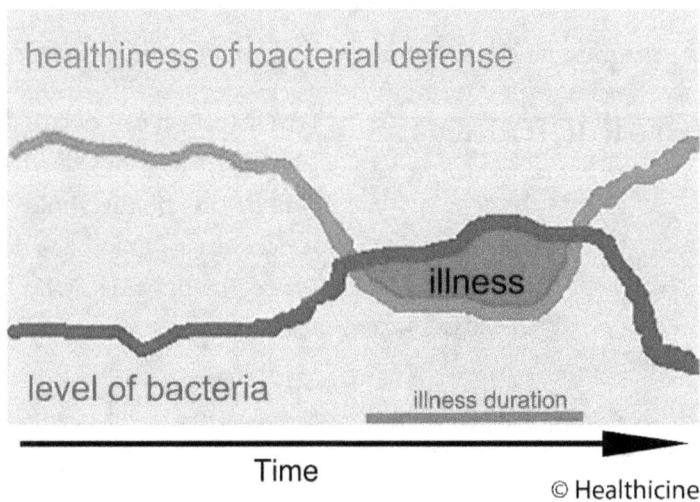

An illness might be a result of both causes. There might be a drop in healthiness of defenses at the same time as a rise in the growth of parasitic bacteria. It can be very difficult to determine the difference between the previous illness cause, and this illness cause. The only proof to be found is in the cure.

Each cause might be connected, a result of the other, and it might be difficult to determine which cause came first. However, which came first is seldom relevant to curing.

In these cases, the illness might be cured by either action or by both actions. When it is cured by improving healthiness, we judge the illness to be caused by the lack of healthiness. When it is cured by a medicine that attacks the bacteria, we say the illness was caused by the bacteria. It's a bit like the particle/wave theory in physics. When we test for a particle, we find the attributes of a particle. When we test for a wave, we find waves.

In cases where both causes are present and causing an illness – there are two illnesses, because two cures are necessary.

The cause that cures is the important cause. The cure is the cause reversed. This might, afterwards, be described (or dismissed) as hindsight bias. However, once a cure is present, there is no need to argue about bias.

When we use two or more actions to cure, we don't know which one worked. But the illness has been cured. We don't need to know. A cure is a cure. It is possible the illness was cured by the patient's health, or by other natural, healthy actions of the patient, irrespective of the treatment used. Using both treatments is more likely to cure – although not the most efficient, not the least expensive and also not the least risk. Medicines are toxic, and treatments with medicines create risk. Treatments with health, when medicines are necessary, can also create risk. Curing is not trivial.

We might have more certainty of the cause by guessing the wrong cause first. When a bacterial infection is treated with an antibiotic, and it keeps returning, the antibiotic is not producing a cure. We need to look at the health of the patient, or the health of the environment. But certainty about cause is less important after a cure.

If the illness recurs or becomes chronic after medical treatment – we need to improve the patient's healthiness. If the illness recurs after we improve the patient's healthiness, either we were not successful in raising the necessary healthiness, or more drastic medical actions are needed.

Unless the illness presents danger to the patient – cures by improving healthiness should be preferred and chosen first. Cures by healthiness contain less risk because they improve the health of the patient. Curing with medicine brings risk. Medicines usually decrease the health of the patient, even if cure.

Curing Deficiency Illness

The absence of or insufficiency of a necessity of health can lead to a hole in healthiness, an illness. In many cases, it takes time for these illnesses to grow to a diagnosable stage. Exceptions, like a deficiency of oxygen, are so dangerous we consider the deficiency to be a danger, not an illness.

Multiple deficiency illnesses can occur at from a single cause. General malnutrition can cause many different deficiency illnesses. We might view some forms of starvation as a meta-deficiency illness. For example, a patient might exhibit symptoms of Vitamin C deficiency, because they are on a starvation diet. Treating them with Vitamin C cannot cure the overall malnutrition illness – and if attempted might only help the patient feel better and even heal better, as other illnesses take over. The cure is to identify the right cause – in this case, a meta-cause, and provide a healthy diet. However, a patient who is suffering from starvation – from a total lack of food, can be considered to be suffering from a single illness element, because it is cured with a single cure action, even though multiple diseases might have been diagnosed.

A deficiency illness can have internal or external causes and causal chains. A patient with scurvy might be suffering from a cook who prepares unhealthy foods, or from an aversion to foods that might prevent scurvy, or from an addiction leading to the total neglect of diet. Which cause is important? The cause that cures. Until the cure is achieved, all causes are speculative.

When the cure is attained, we might argue about the true cause – but these arguments are of little consequence to the case.

Cures for deficiency illnesses are documented in today's medical references, which rarely use the word cure and use is inconsistent when it does occur. The 1950 edition of Merck's Manual of Diagnosis and Treatment suggests supplementation as a cure for infantile scurvy. In this case, supplementation appears to cure because infantile scurvy tends to be temporary. A temporary action suffices. But current medical theory has no definition of a temporary cure. In cases where Vitamin C deficiency is not temporary, supplementation will not cure. It does not address the cause.

Another, less prestigious reference, H. Winter Griffith's Complete Guide to Symptoms, Illness and Surgery, uses the word cure for many nutritional deficiency illnesses stating incorrectly with regards to vitamin deficiencies *"usually curable with vitamin supplementation."* A deficiency illness is cured when the underlying cause is addressed, not when the deficiency is supplemented. With regards to folic acid deficiency it states clearly, and a bit more accurately; *"Usually curable in 2 weeks to 3 months with adequate folic acid intake. It will also depend on the underlying cause."*

Winter Griffith often uses the word cure, while the more authoritative references like MERCK, Lange's, and Harrison's avoid cure. Why do medical references not use the word cure? A skeptic might argue they do not use the word cure because scurvy is cured with a nutrient, a vitamin, not by a medicine, and therefore, scurvy is medically incurable. A belief that cures can only come from a medical professional or a medical treatment is medical chauvinism, not healthy logic.

Others might suggest that these illnesses are not cured, because there is always a risk they will return, and therefore, maybe they're just in remission. Nonsense. Remission is no more scientifically defined than cure. If the cause has not been addressed, the illness has not been cured. If the cause has been addressed, the illness has been cured. When a cause arrives anew – it's a new illness. Unless we clearly define remission as different from cure, we cannot claim *"remission, but not cure."* Remission but not cure is a reduction of signs and symptoms when we know the cause has not been addressed. Cured is when signs and symptoms disappear because the cause has been addressed.

A survey of similar diseases, comparing Winter Griffith's use of cure vs Merck's use of cure provides a different insight. A clear example is constipation. Winter Griffith says *"Constipation may go away on its own. It is usually curable with simple changes in diet or lifestyle."* Merck, on the other hand, devotes many pages to constipation, covering many causes and consequences, but does not use the word cure once. Why the difference? It appears that Merck's authors consider constipation that *"goes away on its own"* to be unimportant, not worthy of coverage. As a result, cures that are simple to Winter Griffith are not documented and not even acknowledged in Merck. Merck's authors are not being malicious; they are simply ignoring conditions that are easily cured. The problem is that, in Merck, cures disappear.

Conventional Medicine Cannot Cure Scurvy

Scurvy is a deficiency disease. It seems strange that conventional medicine does not recommend a cure for scurvy. Wait, didn't we learn how James Lind cured scurvy when we were in grade school? Actually, no. The cure for scurvy, taught in grade school does not cure. Neither does the treatment recommended by conventional medical reference texts. Lind studied scurvy, the causes of scurvy, and even cured scurvy successfully. But James Lind did not study *cure*. His concept and understanding of cure were very weak – and this is no surprise. Today's medical professionals have a similar weakness.

Cured is not defined for scurvy. There is no definition of cured for scurvy in the most, perhaps all authoritative references.

It is important to note that there are two Vitamin C deficiency illnesses, *Vitamin C Deficiency* and *Scurvy,* although medical references do not distinguish well between them. Lind identified three different versions of scurvy, but without attention to cause. The difference has little to do with the dietary cause, being simply differences of severity and duration. Scurvy is rare today, because scurvy requires a prolonged Vitamin C deficiency, which has not been diagnosed and treated, or cured by the natural healthiness of the patient. It takes weeks, sometimes months for symptoms of scurvy to appear even after a total absence of consumption of Vitamin C. On the other hand, Vitamin C deficiency and depletion, according to research published in 2004, ranges from 5 to 23 percent of people, in the USA. By those statistics, somewhere between 16 and 75 million people in the USA suffer from a Vitamin C deficiency.

A causal illness is cured when the cause is addressed. A deficiency illness is cured when the cause of the deficiency is successfully addressed.

Merck, Harrison's, and Lange's recommend treatments to address the signs and symptoms of Vitamin C deficiency and scurvy, but not the cause. They cannot cure, do not cure, and the authors make no claim to cure. Deficiency diseases are *treated.* The word cure is not used – except by lesser authoritative authors.

> *Never attribute to malice that which is adequately explained by stupidity*
> *--- Hanlon's Razor*

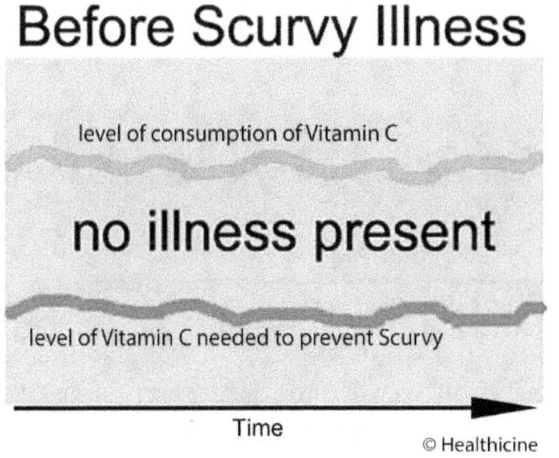

This image shows the normal situation before any Vitamin C deficiency and before scurvy occurs. The person is consuming enough Vitamin C in their diet to prevent the occurrence of a Vitamin C deficiency and to prevent scurvy.

Every deficiency illness, like any causal illness, has two theoretical causes.

1. The consumption of Vitamin C might fall below the amount required to prevent scurvy.
2. The need for Vitamin C might rise above the current consumption of Vitamin C.

Of course, both causes can occur at the same time. The disease scurvy is only diagnosed in the first case and only after the deficiency lasts for weeks. The second case typically occurs as a result of another illness, that increases the need for Vitamin C. It is unlikely to be diagnosed as Vitamin C deficiency because the other illness is more severe.

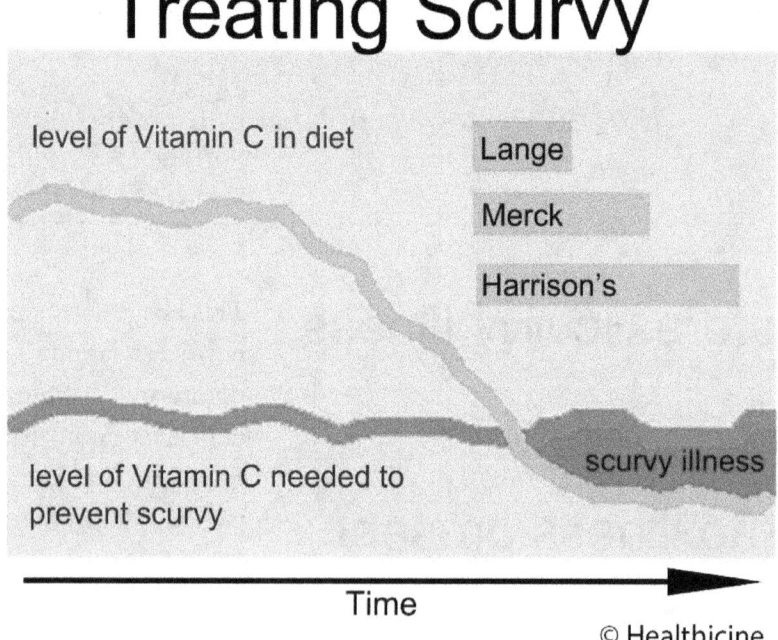

This diagram illustrates what happens when the dietary consumption of Vitamin C drops below the threshold of illness until scurvy can be diagnosed, and the Vitamin C treatments recommended by three major medical reference texts.

Lange's, Merck, and Harrison's recommend different doses of supplemental Vitamin C, for different periods of time, advising that the signs and symptoms of scurvy will quickly disappear. Not one uses the word cure.

Can you see why not? Time marches on. The cause of scurvy is not a lack of medicine, not a lack of Vitamin C supplementation. The cause is an unhealthy diet. Until the diet is changed, the illness is not cured. Signs and symptoms will return shortly after treatment stops. Conventional medical texts consistently recommend a treatment, but not a cure.

Merck, to its credit, also advises: *"followed by a nutritious diet supplying one to two times the daily recommended intake"* but does not specify a duration and does not use the word cure. This action can cure, if it is continued forever – but Merck does not use the word cure and does not recommend forever.

Most deficiency illnesses are causal illnesses, caused by an ongoing absence, so they require healthy cure actions to be maintained, not forever medicines. With causal illnesses, the preventative often becomes the cure.

A cure is present when medicines are no longer required. If a patient needs a medicine, a Vitamin C supplement every day, the illness is being treated, but not cured. Repeated medical treatments with Vitamin C might convert a scurvy illness to chronic scurvy but cannot cure.

What is the cure for scurvy? The patient's dietary processes must be changed to meet the deficiency. The change must be maintained until the patient dies, although by that time – it is no longer a change.

Curing Scurvy

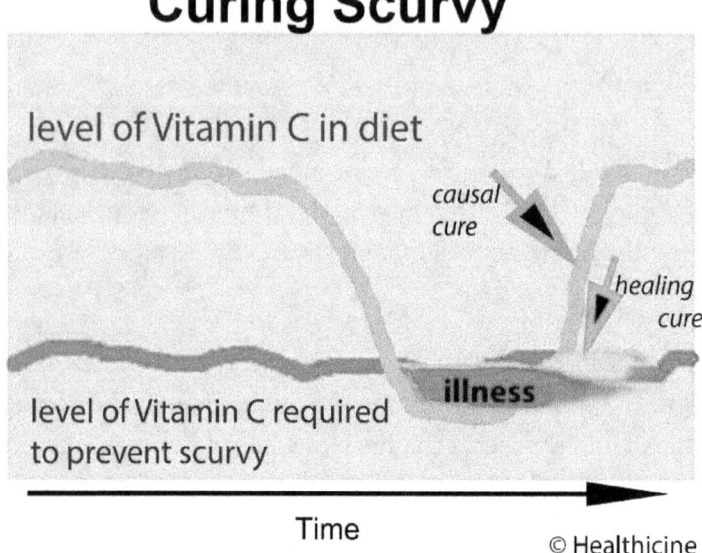

When the level of Vitamin C in the diet rises above the amount required to prevent scurvy, the causal scurvy illness begins to be cured.

After the causal cure, the patient may have injuries caused by scurvy which must be healed. Healing, a second cure, is aided by supplemental Vitamin C, the treatment recommended by medical reference texts. Although medical texts recognize the cause of scurvy as a dietary deficiency of Vitamin C, they only recommend treatments for healing, ignoring the cause. As a result, their treatment recommendations cannot cure scurvy. I suspect the assumption is that any doctor who is treating scurvy will advise the patient of the true cause and expect the patient to address the causal illness. However, this approach results in the disappearance of a cure from medical texts, and a misunderstanding of the cure required and the alternatives possible, unless the doctor reads between the lines.

This might not be a serious problem if scurvy was the only example of this error. However, the same omission occurs again and again in medical reference texts that focus on treatment, while ignoring cure. The result of medical chauvinism is cure blindness.

Scurvy can also be a chronic illness – a fact not mentioned in any current treatment reference – although it was noted by Lind. When this happens, it is only cured when the chronic attribute of the deficiency is addressed.

> *Let food be thy medicine and medicine be thy food.*
> *--- attributed to Hippocrates*

Perhaps Hippocrates did not actually make this statement, often attributed to him. In the time of Hippocrates, the concepts of disease and medicines were very weak by today's standards. There is a difference between a dietary change, and a medicine, even if the medicine is a food. Most medicines don't cure. Most foods, even given as medicines, don't cure any illness. A dietary change is a healthicine, not a medicine. If the patient's diet is suffering from a deficiency, an illness can result. Addressing the deficiency will provide temporary relief. Addressing the cause of the deficiency will cure. Cures are about life, about living, not about taking medicine. If we don't eat, we die of starvation, from the diseases of malnutrition, but eating is not a medicine.

Non-Scurvy, Vitamin C Deficiency

The conventional medical disease diagnostic paradigm to scurvy fails to see the big picture. Scurvy is an illness caused when the consumption of Vitamin C falls far below the daily needs, for a long period. Vitamin C deficiency is the same illness less severe, or over a shorter time period.

There are other situations where the need for Vitamin C rises to a point where normal levels of consumption are not sufficient.

This might be due to another illness, or a toxin in the patient. The online MSD (Merck Sharp & Dohme) Manual says: *"The need for dietary vitamin C is increased by febrile illnesses, inflammatory disorders (particularly diarrheal disorders), achlorhydria, smoking, hyperthyroidism, iron deficiency, cold or heat stress, surgery, burns, and protein deficiency."* Animals create their own Vitamin C. Humans cannot and must handle these situations with consumption of Vitamin C in diet or supplements.

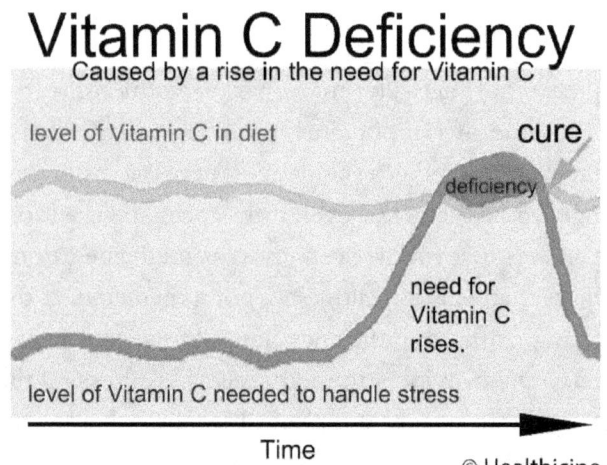

In this diagram, the cure is to address the unhealthiness of the patient, not the unhealthiness of the diet.

Additional dietary or supplementary Vitamin C will aid the cure. If the cause is temporary, supplemental Vitamin C might appear to cure, and be credited with a cure – because the cause goes away as time passes. Sometimes appearing to cure is a cure. In some cases, providing what the body needs to address the unhealthiness provides a cure.

These illnesses and their cures are poorly studied by conventional medicine. A temporary Vitamin C deficiency is not likely to be diagnosed as a disease if another medical condition exists. The conventional medicine focus on diagnosable diseases fails to find the Vitamin C illness and thus fails to understand that cure element. The patient will not develop scurvy, because the increased need is short term. However, these situations can present danger to the health and the life of the patient.

As with a bacterial infection, it is possible for a deficiency illness to emerge from both causes.

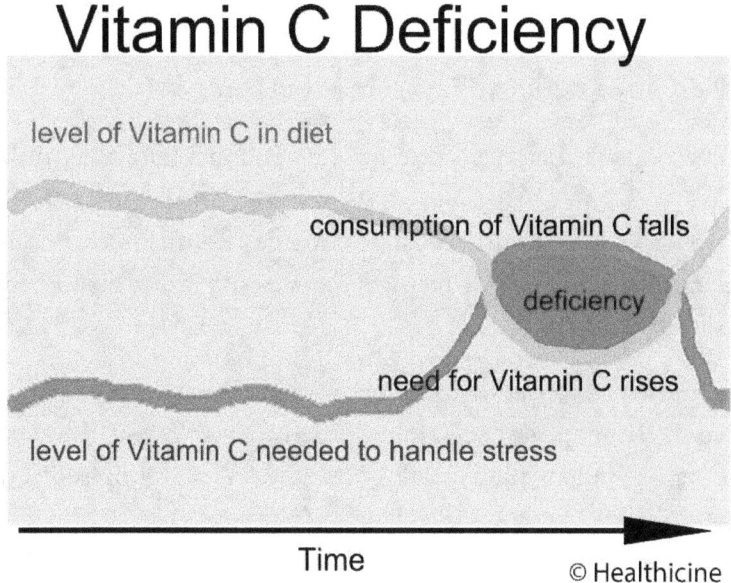

In this diagram, a Vitamin C deficiency emerges when consumption drops, at the same time as a condition increases the need for Vitamin C. Either might occur first. One minor condition, or the other, might exist undetected for some time because, by itself, it might not cause any diagnosable disease. Even when both conditions exist together, the condition might be difficult, even impossible to diagnose in the current conventional medical paradigm, if it is not severe enough for a clear diagnosis. It might be only diagnosed by a cure. This condition can easily recur even become chronic if the consumption of Vitamin C remains low after the stress is addressed. Supplemental Vitamin C temporarily addresses one cause, but not the other. It might appear to cure, but the cure will not last unless the other conditions change. There are two illnesses, because two cures are needed.

This type of illness, with two causes acting together, is a challenge for current medical practice, which does not study cause in individual cases of a disease. Over the short term, it might be diagnosed as increased severity of one illness, rather than two separate illnesses. If it continues over the long term, it is labelled chronic. If it does not reach the level required for a diagnosis of scurvy, it might be judged, diagnosed as a mystery chronic illness – incurable – because we don't understand. We understand less when we aim to treat, but not to cure.

Maybe you've noticed that, according to conventional medicine, most diseases have *multiple contributing factors.* The phrase multiple contributing factors is often an excuse to provide treatments that don't cure. Looking for, finding, and recognizing cures is impossible in the current medical paradigm.

An illness with two causes consists of two illness elements. If an illness with two causal elements is successfully treated for one cause, the signs and symptoms will fade. The illness – one illness – is still present but might be invisible. The patient will feel better. This looks like an effective treatment. Later, when a similar cause arrives a new illness occurs, but is perceived as a reemergence or increase in severity of the same "disease". In the treatment paradigm, it looks like a remission and recurrence. It was a successful cure element, a partial cure, followed by a new occurrence of a cause, leading to a new occurrence of an illness element.

What is the true cause? What is the cure? When there are *two contributing causes*, in many cases, addressing one or the other will provide a cure. If the condition is temporary, any action might appear to cure, as the illness is cured by health. Addressing both causes improves the probability of success, while improving the healthiness of the patient. The wrong treatment, supplemental Vitamin C, might appear to be successful from a short-term measurement of signs and symptoms, as it fails to cure the longer-term illness. Most clinical studies are short term. Most clinical studies don't define cured and don't test for cured.

When there are two or more elements of illness present, it is necessary to address two or more causes to cure. Two or more cures are required.

This might even occur with two causes of a single deficiency illness. A person with two causes of Vitamin C deficiency illness has two illnesses, requiring two cures, one for each cause. For example, an alcoholic, who suffers a vitamin deficiency because they prefer alcohol over food and also suffers from extreme poverty will not be cured by removing either single cause. If the alcoholism is cured, they will still be too poor to buy healthy food. If the poverty is cured, they might spend the money on alcohol, not food. Two causes exist, two illnesses exist, and two cures are necessary, even though it might be diagnosed as a single disease.

The cure identifies the cause. If we increase the dietary consumption of Vitamin C, and there is no cure, we must search for another cause. If there is a cure, that was the cause. If we reduce a stress, and that action cures, the cure identifies the cause. Once we aim to cure, once we take action with an aim to cure, there is less confusion. Confusion grows when we fail to aim for a cure, when we only treat signs and symptoms, permitting causes to continue and illness to persist and grow.

Chronic Non-Scurvy Vitamin C Deficiency

It is possible, to have a situation where the level of consumption of Vitamin C is low – but not low enough to lead to a diagnosis of Vitamin C deficiency or scurvy. A chronic, non-disease level deficiency of Vitamin C. This condition might exist for years, even decades without any diagnosis. It can lead to creeping chronic conditions, difficult to diagnose, impossible to cure in medical theory. This type of low-level illness can happen with many other deficiencies – not just nutrient deficiencies. A patient might also suffer multiple minor non-diagnosable nutrient deficiencies which together create serious health problems – but little possibility of a diagnosis, because no named disease exists. When conventional medical practice encounters these cases, it often finds success in treating signs and symptoms. Treating signs and symptoms *works* even when it cannot cure.

Cures can be found – when we look for cures.

Deficiency or Excess?

We can view every illness as caused by a deficiency of healthiness. We can view every illness as caused by an excess of stress. A deficiency of healthiness is stressful. An excess of stress is a deficiency of healthiness.

There are, as previously discussed, significant differences between illnesses caused by deficiencies and illnesses caused by stress, and it is important to be conscious of these differences when aiming to cure.

Deficiency illnesses are always in waiting. A deficiency cause is present when the necessary is absent. Each deficiency illness element has a single deficiency cause, although each case has different causal chains. Many deficiency illnesses are generic – the same deficiency in a different person will have very similar consequences, timelines, prognoses and cures. Different patients will suffer the same illness from a severe deficiency of Vitamin C, although the signs and symptoms of several deficiencies occurring together might be very unclear and varied from one person to another, because every illness depends on the healthiness of the patient.

Treating signs and symptoms can put a deficiency illness into remission, but it cannot cure. Treating a deficiency directly might also put the illness into remission, but rarely leads to a cure. The illness will return when the treatment is stopped unless a natural cure occurs.

Deficiency illnesses are cured when the cause of the deficiency is addressed. Another deficiency illness, not a remission, occurs if the cause recurs, or if the same deficiency occurs due to a different cause. When an attribute of the deficiency cause is chronic, the illness will not be cured until the chronic nature of the cause is addressed.

The opposite of a deficiency illness is an illness of excess. We often use the word stress to describe the cause of an illness caused by an excess of something. We might view a deficiency illness as *a stress,* but illnesses caused by excess have a different nature, different causes, and require different types of cures. Deficiency illnesses are cured by adding or increasing something, excess-caused-illnesses are cured by removing reducing something. Illnesses caused by lack of exercise, like some cases of arthritis and bedsores, might be considered stress illnesses because the cause is an *absence of healthy stress,* but they can only be cured by adding something – physical exercise, so they are deficiency illnesses.

The severity of an illness of excess depends not just on the stress, but also on the healthiness and strength of the patient. Stress illnesses can vary widely from individual to individual, depending on the strength of the stress, on the strength of the individual, and other stresses they are experiencing. Physical deficiency illnesses are often more consistent in their consequences. Deficiencies of mind, spirits, or community are less consistent in consequences because the patient's health is often supported by other factors.

Every illness, whether caused by a deficiency or an excess, can be incidental if the cause is a single event, repeating if the cause and cure repeat several times, or chronic if the cause persists or repeats continually over time.

Curing Illness caused by Excesses

Stress is essential to life. We walk by falling, then recovering in a new position. Without the stress and risk of falling, we cannot move forward. Illness can be caused by excessive stress. What is excessive? An amount that causes illness.

Excessive stress might be physical stress, leading to injuries, broken bones, or nutritional stress, leading to many different types of illness, or stress on the mind, leading to poor life decisions, or stress on the spirit, leading to poor or unhealthy motivation, or stress on the communities, leading to illnesses of community – which are often classified and diagnosed as illnesses of the mind, and then treated with chemicals for the body.

An excess might exist in a process, like consumption of food, in injuries due to over-exercising, or excesses of attributes from fat to fear. Many necessaries become stresses in excess. Vitamins are essential nutrients, but too much can lead to illness.

Illnesses caused by excesses can be cured by improving the patient's strength and health such that the excess can be tolerated, or by reducing the level of the excess. The cure proves the cause. It can be important to find the cause that provides the best cure.

Excesses can also cause injuries, which require healing. When an excessive stress is in the past, the illness is an injury illness, not a causal illness. We might blame the cause but addressing it will not cure, even though it may prevent future cases. Injury illnesses need to be healed. When the excess that caused an injury is also present, two illnesses are present, and two cures necessary.

Sometimes medicine improves a patient's ability to ignore the stress of an excess. Sometimes they give a patient time to recover strength, such that their healthiness provides a cure. Medicines can also make the patient feel stronger by numbing sensitivity, creating an illusion of helping without any attempt to address the cause, without any attempt to cure, giving the patient an ability to tolerate higher levels of excess causing more damage, leading to more injuries, even to chronic injuries and other illnesses.

Illnesses Caused by Excessive Stress

Causal illnesses caused by excessive stress can emerge when stress rises too high, or when the ability to tolerate or make use of stress falls too low. When the ability to handle a stress falls, it might be due to an increasing number of stresses. We have a finite ability to handle a variety of stresses, and this ability varies over time, hourly, daily, weekly, monthly, seasonally, and as we age.

A stress illness might be caused by internal or external forces. In many cases, illnesses caused by stress are chronic, because the cause is chronic. If the cause is not chronic, the illness might be an injury – a broken bone, a wound, a bruise of body, harm to mind, spirit, or community, that needs to be healed. Stress is a force, sometimes an attribute of a job, a relationship, or some other factor. Stress can lead to negative attributes, causing an attribute illness.

Viewpoint informs judgement about illness. A patient suffering from a chronic repetitive stress injury might view the illness as caused by their job, or their environment, while a friend, boss, or community see it as caused by their unwillingness to change jobs, to change the way the work is done, or a lack of awareness of what is the cause. While the patient, friends, and physicians debate the cause, the illness can grow. The patient wants a cure from the doctor, who cannot change the patient's situation or actions. The doctor can offer treatments for symptoms, but not cures. So, the patient buys a treatment, a symptomicine. Medical insurance pays for approved treatments, regardless of whether they cure, or not. The cause can only be proven with a cure. When an employee is fired, an illness might be cured. When the employee retires, or finds a new job, an illness might be cured. In each case, there is little point in arguing the cause. A patient who claims a change of job cured their illness might be told: *"That's just anecdotal evidence."* Every cure is an anecdote. Some cures, like loss of employment, might be undesirable even as they cure. But until a cure is found, the illness persists and grows.

As with deficiency illnesses, conventional medicine does not define cured for any illnesses caused by excessive exposure to a stressor. There is no testable cure for carbon monoxide poisoning, nor for obesity –

unhealthy food consumption, nor any illness caused by excessive physical, mental, emotional, spirit, or community stress. Conventional medicine offers treatments for these illnesses. Cured is not defined and cannot be proven scientifically even after an illness is cured.

The healthicine model for stress caused illness is generic. It covers stresses caused by toxic chemicals, stress caused by toxic habits, stress caused by toxic levels of consumption of normally health substances. Because stress is such a general term, this model might be used for any causal illness, even a deficiency illness, with appropriate changes to labels. It is conceptually identical to the model used for excessive growth of bacteria – a bacterial stress.

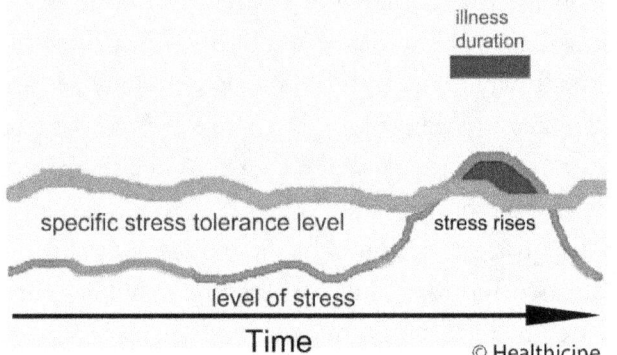

In this diagram, the person can handle a specific stress in their life, until the stress increases in severity.

We might experience excessive stress from and in the diet, body, mind, spirit, or community. The stresses of a bacterial infection and the stresses that cause a broken arm are physical. The stress of too many tasks, too many things to remember is mental. The stress of loss of job, loss of identity, loss of incentive is a stress on our spirits. We might experience community stress from excessive responsibilities, or excessive reliance on others.

When a stress overcomes a person's stress tolerance, a stress illness can occur. The cure is to address the stress or sometimes to raise the levels of strength and healthiness, of stress tolerance, to handle the stress without illness.

Illness Caused by Deficiency of Stress Tolerance

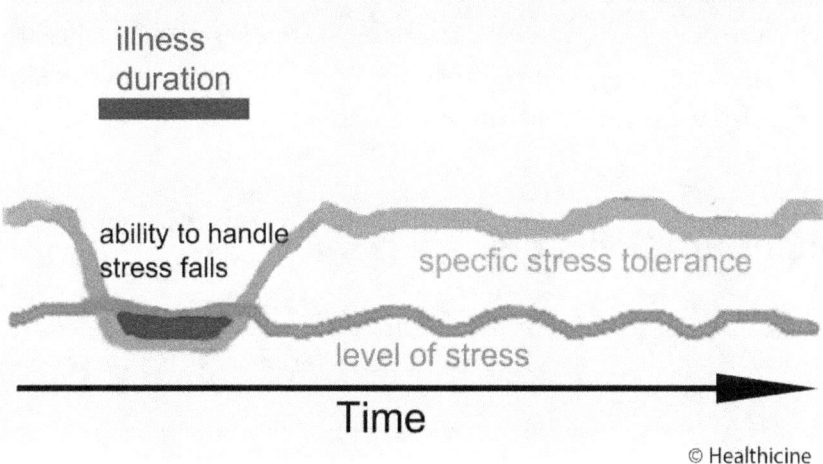

The same disease, diagnosed using only signs and symptoms, can emerge from another cause, a drop in healthiness, as in this diagram.

As a person's healthiness, their ability to handle a specific stress drops below the current level of stress, and a stress illness occurs. This illness is cured when healthiness rises above the level of stress, giving relief, facilitating recovery and healing. Raising healthiness can be hard.

The signs and symptoms of this case can be identical to an illness caused by an excess of stress. Patients might be treated with the same medicine, a symptomicine. But the illnesses have different causes and require different cures. The first requires a reduction in stress; the second requires an improvement in the healthiness of the patient. An incorrect or incomplete diagnosis and treatment, that does not cure, that can lead to chronic stress illness.

As with deficiency illnesses, it is possible to have a stress illness with both causes – a drop in tolerance for a specific stress and a rise in the same stress. With stress caused illnesses, there is another complication; each stress lowers our ability to deal with stress, increasing the potential for stress illnesses.

Every illness, when not cured, can cause more illnesses. We might claim that stress illnesses are most likely to cause other illnesses. However, every cause of illness can be viewed as a stress. Every stress has a healthy level (sometimes zero) and an unhealthy level, which can vary for each individual and as their life situation changes.

Other Cure Concepts

> *Faith does not make things easy,*
> *It makes them possible.*
> *--- Luke 1:37*

Although conventional medicine does not define and does not study cures, practitioners and pundits spend a lot of time dismissing cure claims. Cure claims for most diseases are ignored. Conventional medicine places more faith in not-cures than in cures. Faith in the incurability of an illness can make cures impossible. Faith in cures makes them possible, but as the Bible advises, faith does not make things easy.

Spirit Cures: The Power of Intention

Spirits are intentions. Our intentions depend on faith, on what we believe is possible. Faith determines what is possible. Intentions can cure many illness, when intentions drive healthy actions. Sometimes they even determine what happened. When we believe we can, we prove we can. When we believe we cannot, we easily prove ourselves right.

When our doctor's spirits and ours are not aligned, something may need to change before we can find a cure. A patient might say *"it only hurts when I do this,"* and the doctor might advise *"then, don't do that."* The patient can choose to agree with the doctor or not, or perhaps to find a different doctor.

Spirits are real. Intention is a spirit, a reality, not a placebo. If we decide our illness is curable, but our doctor believes it is incurable, we might be on our own, until we find a doctor – or someone else - who believes in cures. If we cure our illness, our doctor might even deny the cure, or more likely, accept the cure, while denying a specific cause of the cure. Medical doctors have no training a cure. They are experienced with cure uncertainty, can practice denial, but not validation.

Sometimes our doctor believes our illness is curable – when we believe it is incurable. Sometimes a patient denies that a cure has been accomplished. Cured is a judgement, not a fact. Belief is essential to cure.

Placebo Cures

> *A beneficial effect produced by a placebo drug or treatment, which cannot be attributed to the properties of the placebo itself, and must therefore be due to the patient's belief in that treatment.*
> Oxford Dictionary

Can placebos cure? Yes. Can a placebo effect be a cure? No.

It's important to separate placebo from placebo effect. As Oxford's definition above clearly states, placebo effects are NOT caused by the placebo. The Oxford dictionary *sample sentence* for placebo effect is telling: "*orthodox doctors dismiss the positive results as a result of the placebo effec*t." The phrase placebo effect is generally used to dismiss positive results. No placebo effect can be a cure. Many researchers propose hypothetical causes of placebo effects – and there is general agreement that placebo effects cannot be cures.

Sometimes when health cures – especially if the patient has taken an alternative medicine, conventional medicine claims it's *"only a placebo effect."* Placebo effect is in the dictionary, but not *placebo cure*. Placebo effects, like most medical treatments, cannot cure.

Placebos, on the other hand, are not so restricted. We often think of a placebo as a null medicine or treatment, but placebos cover a much wider span of treatments. Many clinical study placebos are designed to have real effects, to mimic the drug being tested – but not the benefits. In addition, many alternative treatments are dismissed as placebos. But they are real treatments, and sometimes they cure. Placebos can cure. Because placebos have real effects – they can sometimes cure. There have been several clinical studies, I have seen at least two, where the placebo arm of the trial produced cures. However, most clinical trials do not test for cures, so in most cases – when a cure occurs in either arm of the clinical trial, the cure is ignored. When a placebo cures, the cure is ignored. When a conventional medical treatment cures, the cure is also often ignored. When health cures, the cure is ignored.

Placebo effects, by definition, are not caused by the treatment, although the definition is illogical: *"an improvement in the condition of the patient that occurs* **in response to a treatment** *but* **cannot be considered due to the specific treatment** *used"* (Webster). By definition: a paradox. Most of what is written about placebo effects is scientific nonsense, a result of the paradox.

There is no doubt, no disagreement about the beneficial nature of placebo effects. A placebo effect is a real, positive effect *where the doctor does not believe the treatment caused the effect*. In that sense, placebo effects are caused by the doctor (or the disbelief of the doctor). Every effect has a cause.

Placebo effect can only be claimed when we do not understand the cause. If we understand the cause, it's a real effect, with a real cause. If we don't understand the cause, it's a real effect, with a real cause that we do not understand. Calling it a placebo effect does not help us understand the cause. It's a deliberate technique to ignore the cause. Every effect has a cause. Every cause has a cause. Every cause of a cause has a cause. Every cause is part of a chain of causes, which we can extend forever. Just as every illness has a chain of causes, every improvement has a chain of causes.

A so-called *placebo effect* is only one link in a causal chain. Once we understand the cause, once we endeavor to study the causal chain, it's no longer a placebo effect. However, once *placebo effect* is claimed, we stop investigating the chain of causes. Most placebo effects are statistical, a result of clinical studies, not actual cases. This distracts us from cures.

Most placebo effects are treatment effects, but not cures. Most placebos, like most medicines, are symptomicines – affecting only signs and symptoms.

"Expectation is a form of mind cure."
Ted Kaptchuk

Ted J. Kaptchuk, a placebo effect researcher, writes in the New England Journal of Medicine *"placebo effects are improvements in patients' symptoms that are attributable to their participation in the therapeutic encounter, with its rituals, symbols, and interactions."* This makes no sense. Why call them placebo effects, if we know the cause? We should call them effects of *"participation in the therapeutic encounter,"* or *"its rituals,"* or *"its symbols,"* or *"its interactions,"* and study each in turn.

> *"Sham treatments cannot shrink tumors or cure viruses."*
> Ted Kaptchuk

Ted Kaptchuk claims, and the American Cancer Society agrees: "placebo effects cannot shrink tumors" without providing any evidence. But a simple search of PubMed shows clinical trials where the placebo arm shows tumors to be diminished, sometimes by more than the drug being tested.

Jo Merchant, in the book Cure: A Journey into the Science of Mind over Body claims *"A rigorous, skeptical, deeply reported look at the new science behind the mind's surprising ability to heal the body,"* but does not define heal and does not define cure. Instead, it refers only to cure *claims* and *bogus-cures*. Without a scientific definition of cure, how can we claim to be rigorous? Suggesting that a cure is a placebo effect is resorting to medical mysticism, to explain away what we don't understand.

Recognized cures are not called placebo effects. Most cures are not recognized. Many cures are referred to as placebo effects without any attempt at validation of the claim.

> *"The one thing of which we can be absolutely certain is that placebos do not cause placebo effects. Placebos are inert and don't cause anything."*
> Daniel Moerman, Deconstructing the Placebo Effect and Finding the Meaning Response *2002.*

Unfortunately, Daniel Moerman then went on to explain placebo effects as the *meaning response.* Meaning can be manipulated, and that manipulated meaning can be a treatment causing the meaning response. If meaning response is a real cause of a real effect – then it is not a placebo effect. It is a link in the causal chain. What caused that link?

If changing the patient's mind, or changing the patient's belief, or faith, truly produces a cure, the lack of faith was the cause. The cure proves the cause. If they are cured by a change in their belief in the doctor, the medicine or treatment, they have been cured by community, not by a medicine, not by a placebo.

Cures are caused by health, by improving healthiness. Placebo cures are also caused by health. The mistake of dismissing benefits and cures we do not understand to *"the mind"* or to the *"beliefs of the patient"* is mystical nonsense.

It's not hard to understand why conventional medicine so often resorts, even embraces, placebo effect explanations. Conventional medicine has little ability to recognize, and less ability to understand causes of the mind, the spirits, or the communities of a patient. In addition, conventional medicine has little interest in recognizing effectiveness of alternative treatments, which would be a hole in the damn, releasing a flood of acknowledgment that non-conventional treatments can provide benefits, even cure. Placebo effect is a ready excuse, always at hand, seldom questioned or investigated. Investigation might find a true cause, and a true cause is not a placebo, by definition. So cases labelled placebo effects are dismissed, never investigated. Instead, they are studied statistically, where nothing can be proven in any single case.

Can placebos cure? Yes. We need to look at each of type of cure in turn. There are three types of illness, causal, injury, and attribute illnesses and the three associated types of cures.

Placebos cannot cure a causal illness. A causal cure must be maintained to maintain the cure. If a placebo treatment must be maintained to maintain the cure, it's not a placebo, it's an action necessary to the health of the patient.

Placebos cannot cure an injury illness. Injuries are cured by healing. A placebo might help the patient heal, but it cannot cure.

Many placebos are inert. But not all. Some so-called placebos can have powerful effects that can lead to transformation of some aspect of the patient. Also, the act of prescribing the placebo, of believing in the placebo, of believing in the cure, can create a transformation that cures. When these happen, a placebo can cure attribute illnesses. Are there any real-world examples? Yes, of course. But as long as we maintain the mysticism around placebos and placebo effects, these remain invisible.

Placebos can cure attribute illness, by bringing about real change. There are clinical trials where cures occurred on the placebo arm of the trial. However, to my knowledge, no researchers dared document that the placebo *cured* the patient. Why not? There are two main reasons. First of all, researchers are conditioned to believe that placebos can't cure. So, if a cure occurs, it is assumed to be *not* caused by the placebo. Second, most clinical trials measure benefits in signs and symptoms, but do not test for cured, so when cures occur on either arm, they are simply ignored.

Most placebo effects documented and studied are effects on the signs and symptoms of a disease. Most medicines only affect the signs and symptoms of the disease being treated – so it's natural to compare placebo treatments to medical treatments using the same *non-curative* standard. As a result, most cures – caused by medicines or by placebo treatments – disappear.

Regression to the Mean

Another rationalization presented against improvements in signs and symptoms, even of cures, attributed to alternative treatments is *regression to the mean.*

Regression to the mean is a statistical observation, not a cause. Actual cures have actual causes. Every instance of improvement or cure attributed to regression to the mean has a real cause, not a statistical cause.

When an anecdotal cure (all cures are anecdotes), or an improvement (all improvements have causes) in the patient's condition is attributed to *"regression to the mean,"* it's a nonsense claim. There is no *mean* in a single case. Without a statistical measure of mean in a group of cases, we cannot know if any individual case is regressing to the mean, or improving faster than the mean, or improving or moving in a different direction from the mean. Regression to the mean is useful to explain statistical results, but not to explain individual results. Every individual result is an anecdote, not a statistic, a unique, individual story.

Miracle Cures

Do miracle cures exist? What is a miracle cure?

The book **Miracle Cures: Saints, Pilgrimage, and the Healing Powers of Belief,** by Robert A Scott is an in-depth exploration of the history, and the reality of miracle cures. What did Robert A Scott learn?

First of all, we need to understand that Scott does not have a clear definition of cure, nor of miracle, and often uses the word *healing* as a cure, even when the cure appears to have been brought about by causal processes or by transformation. He does have a strong belief that some claims of miracle cures have significant validity saying: *"I argue that the faithful feel confident in appealing to the saints for cures because for certain conditions, and under certain circumstances, such appeals actually work."* Scott does not define *cure* nor *works*. However, the book makes it clear that *works* has more meaning than is generally given in conventional medicine – where works (although seldom articulated as such) generally means *"makes the patient or doctor feel better about their disease but does not cure."*

Scott offers an important caution, with *"I am scarcely the first to point out why a pilgrimage might contribute to a sick person's sense of well being. Changes in diet, climate, and daily routine while travelling to pilgrimage shrines might all have beneficial effects together with the powerful experience of being with others with a common purpose."* There are many possibilities for non-miracle cures. A pilgrimage can improve healthiness. Improved healthiness often cures.

When thousands of people make a pilgrimage to a saint or shrine, each of them changes their diet, their exercise routines, their communities. They develop an individual purpose and a common purpose with the people around them. With so many changes, many cures can be caused by health, by healthy actions. When one person experiences a miraculous cure – the story is repeated and magnified as time passes. Hundreds who die are ignored. The death of a pilgrim is not newsworthy.

> *If you don't believe in miracles,*
> *You could be taking bad advice.*
> *Roy Forbes – Tender Lullaby*

Many cases of a miracle cures can be explained with a relatively simple understanding of the three types of illness and three types of cures. A pilgrimage to a holy shrine affects the health of diet, body, mind, spirit, and community, sometimes positively, sometimes negatively, and can produce illness or cures without clear intention. If someone makes a pilgrimage to a shrine for a cure and finds themselves cured, they are not likely to give credit to their dietary changes, changes to their daily exercise routines, changes to their mental status and their spirits, their sense of purpose. The credit goes to the saint, to the shrine. That's why they went on the pilgrimage.

Scott comments on the lack of scientific evidence of cures: *"biomedical and other scientists need to understand that despite the complete absence of independently verifiable, quantitative empirical data about the physical ailments afflicting visitors to medieval shrines....,"* but fails to recognize that many of today's illnesses are mental, spirit, and community illnesses, which do not provide *"independently verifiable quantitative empirical data"* to researchers – because these illnesses, their causes, and their cures are not recognized by conventional medicine. Conventional medicine blindly views all illnesses as physical realities of the body.

Scott also fails to recognize that there is no science of cure today. In Chapter five, he comments about epidemiology, with *"No studies of medieval illness employ modern standards of epidemiology."* But epidemiology does not study cures. Cure is intentionally not defined in dictionaries of epidemiology. *"Epidemiology is more interested in the prevention and control of disease than secondary and tertiary curative approaches found in traditional medicine."* Thomas C Timmreck, Ph.D. states in **An Introduction to Epidemiology**, 2nd Edition. There is no science of medicine today that studies cures. Cures are not defined for most diseases and cannot be studied scientifically as a result. Conventional medical science uses powerful and persuasive arguments to dismiss cures – but has no tools to validate cures at all – except for a few communicable diseases cured by poisonous medicines.

Can miracles cure? Do miracle cures exist? Every cure is a miracle when we fail to understand cause of illness and the associated cure.

Zipless Cures

Conventional medicine is searching for zipless cures, cures that are absolutely pure, single chemicals, patentable, free of side effects.

Cures that do the job and leave quietly.

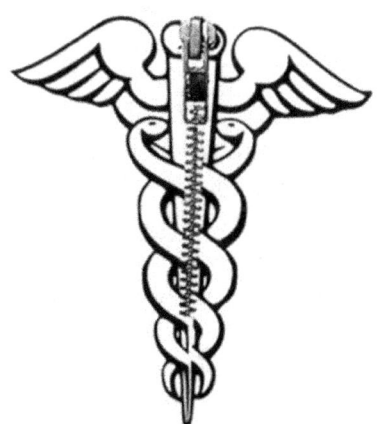
© Healthicine

But, zipless cures are rarer than unicorns.

In 1973, Eric Jong wrote in Fear of Flying: *"The zipless fuck is absolutely pure. It is free of ulterior motives. There is no power game... No one is trying to prove anything or get anything out of anyone. The zipless fuck is the purest thing there is. And it is rarer than the unicorn."*

The business of medicine wants zipless cures.

Ziploss cures are efficient and easy. They don't require complex analysis, no need for a relationship between the physician and the patient. The diagnosis is completed, the physician prescribes the treatment, the patient takes the treatment, never to return. Zipless.

Health and illness are not zipless. Health is about life, constantly changing until we die. The health of an individual is about their life, their activities, their habits, their relationships, their communities and their environment. Illnesses are also about the life of the patient.

There are three types of diseases according to the World Health Organization, published in the ICD10 – the International Classification of Diseases:
- communicable diseases, HIV, TB, etc.
- non-communicable diseases: hypertension, breast cancer, etc.

- external causes of injuries: traffic accident, drowning.

Injuries

No medicine can cure an injury. Injuries are only cured by health and healing. Symptomicines are medicines that mask the symptoms of injury.

Communicable Diseases

Medicine is searching for zipless cures for communicable diseases like the common cold, pneumonia, HIV and Tuberculosis. We might want to believe antibiotics, antifungal, and antiviral medicines are zipless, but the more we use them, the more we learn their risks and potential problems. Medicines that fight and kill unhealthy living organisms also fight and kill healthy living organisms in our bodies and our environments. Bacteria and other parasites evolve. Medicines that kill only work for a short time, sometimes prompting the evolution of a more dangerous organism. Evolution can be pushed forward, to a state dangerous to our health, by the not-zipless cure – which kills off the original, less harmful even beneficial, bacterial competitor.

Preventatives

Conventional medicine is also searching for zipless preventatives. Vaccines and fluoride are often presented as zipless preventatives, working perfectly, free of risk. Every preventative action has a cost-benefit ratio, which can change over time. Preventions that improve healthiness have more benefits and less risks. Every preventative measure presents risks that need to be studied. There is no serious interest in the study of cost-benefit, nor of risk, in the prevention industries. There is only the denial of risk. All preventative medicines need to be zipless for marketing purposes.

When you get the common cold, is it your fault? It's not difficult to blame the patient, in fact, it's commonplace. You shouldn't go out in the cold. You should have worn a sweater. You should wash your hands. Blame is all around us. Your doctor doesn't want to blame you for your cold, although, if you blame yourself, they might agree - to help you feel better. The cold needs to be treated. It needs to be cured. Conventional medicine wants a zipless cure for the common cold, a cure that zips in and gets rid of the cold, without putting any responsibility on the patient, without any responsibility on the doctor – except to sign the prescription. A zipless cure for the common cold would be a best-seller. There is a cure for the common cold. The cure for the common cold is trivial. It has been described, accurately, by Darrell Huff: *"Proper treatment will cure a cold in seven days, but left to itself, a cold will hang on for a week."* The cure for the common cold is health.

But when we have a cold, or any illness – we want a cure, a zipless cure.

Non-Communicable Diseases

Conventional medicine is also searching for zipless cures for non-communicable diseases like hypertension, diabetes, breast cancers, arthritis, and obesity. But this is an error in understanding.

An illness can only be cured by addressing the cause. We can't kill the cause of obesity, or hypertension. The cause is an absence of healthiness. These illnesses can only be cured with health, not with medicines. Health is not zipless. Improving healthiness requires commitment. If a doctor or the medical establishment wants to cure these illnesses – they need to commit to a relationship with the patient, not to zipless cures.

Many illnesses are caused by the actions of the patient, perhaps more by the non-activities of the patient. Obesity is caused, in theory, by eating too much, or by the absence of restraint. Scurvy is caused, in theory, by not eating enough Vitamin C. But in practice, none of these causes lead us directly to cures. Finding cure causes, finding real cures, is challenging work, not zipless. Conventional medicine searches for zipless cures for every illness. But zipless cures are rarer than unicorns. What can be done? There are two solutions in common use today.

Cure Avoidance

Conventional medicine avoids the word cure, preferring incurable. The common cold is incurable. Obesity is incurable. Depression is incurable. All mental disorders are incurable. Heart disease is incurable. Diseases caused by viruses are incurable. Chronic diseases are incurable. Conventional medicine has given up searching for cures because it wants zipless cures – which do not exist. So, what to do?

Zipless Treatments

Conventional medicine searches instead for zipless therapies and zipless treatments, for treatments that don't cure. Treatments are good for the economy. We buy insurance. Insurance pays for treatments. We pay again. Our insurance pays again. Everybody benefits. Treatments are a growth business.

Treatments and therapies provide many (economic) benefits over cures:

- treatments can be tested in clinical studies, documented as such, presented as scientific, and approved by government agencies.
- treatments carry no guarantee. It's accepted that they don't cure, even that they don't work at all in many cases,
- they can be patented and manufactured, bought and sold,
- they are provided by a doctor, not based on changing the patient, not based on a relationship between doctor and patient,
- it's easy to prove a treatment works. The definition of works for a treatment is generally *"has beneficial effect on some signs and symptoms, and adverse consequences, or side effects, but does not cure,"*

- no-one expects a treatment to cure, or we would call it a cure,
- when a drug patent expires, it's easy to find a new drug, after all, it doesn't need to cure,
- treatments sometimes have some severe negative effects without significant market repercussions. We expect side effects from treatments,

Curing, on the other hand, is harder, cures cannot be tested in clinical studies because cured is not defined most diseases.

> *I do not mean to say that lemon juice and wine are the only remedies for the scurvy ; this disease, like many others, may be cured by medicines of very different and opposite qualities to each other, and to that of lemons.*
> *James Lind, A Treatise on Scurvy, 1771*

There are many unique cures for a simple disease like scurvy, which is treated as incurable in current medical reference texts.

The preference for treatments and therapies over cures can be seen in the titles of major medical reference texts:
- MERCK Manual of Diagnosis and **Therapy**
- Lange's Current Medical Diagnosis and **Treatment**
- Harrison's **Principles** of Internal Medicine: Disease Parthenogenesis and **Treatment**
- **Diagnostic** and **Statistical** Manual of Mental Disorders

Not one of these references contains a definition of cure. They occasionally use the word cure, although not consistently. Individual sections are written by different authors, who have no standard scientific definition of cure, there being no medical definition nor test for most disease cures. Cure, understood by many schoolchildren and grandmothers, is not defined medically nor scientifically. Most diseases have become incurable, by lack of definition. If a mental disease has a curable cause – then it's not a mental disease, it's caused by the cause.

A treatment prolongs an illness. It reduces symptoms and helps us to live with the illness, to live longer with the illness. In doing so, it helps the illness to live longer as well. Treatments that do not cure create chronic illnesses – a market for more treatments. Treatments are more financially successful than cures. There are powerful economic incentives to develop, test, and market treatments over cures.

Chronic Treatments

We shouldn't be surprised so many diseases are chronic. While we search for zipless cures – finding only treatments, we also find chronic treatments, which can convert curable illnesses to chronic diseases.

A cure cures. When an illness is cured, it's gone. No further treatments, no further medicines are required. Cures trump treatments.

Even the recommended treatment for scurvy is not zipless. If you have an illness caused by a nutritional deficiency, or dietary toxicity, or sleep deficiency, or exercise excess, cured is not defined. Medical reference texts occasionally suggest that meeting the deficiency over the short term is a cure – a simple misunderstanding of the concept of cured.

No one pretends the recommended treatment for scurvy is a zipless cure. If we give the patient ascorbic acid, synthetic Vitamin C, the symptoms of scurvy will go away. As soon as the treatment is discontinued, the illness returns. More medicine, more ascorbic acid addresses the symptoms. Although not recognized by medical authorities, ascorbic acid, the treatment recommended by all major references, can only create a chronic illness, requiring chronic treatment. The same is true of sleeping pills for sleep deficiency and many other recommended treatments.

Scurvy can only be cured by health. Health is not zipless. Health is the best medicine, the best cure.

The Perfect Cure Myth

> "Psychotherapy does not cure patients; rather it helps them to change. Cure implies that the problem will never recur - a questionable claim for any healing profession."
> *The Textbook of Psychotherapeutic Treatments*

Nonsense. Cures are not perfect. An illness is not something that can go away and return. Recurrence is not a return of the illness that left or faded away.

Medical professionals often feel the need to cure now – and in the future as well. We can only cure a present illness, by addressing a present cause. An illness element is cured when the present cause has been addressed. If you have a bacterial infection and you cure it with an antibiotic that kills the bacteria, it's a cure. It can be tested and proven as a cure. If you are exposed to the bacteria, the cause, again, you get a new infection, not a remission. That's how cures work.

If someone has a mental illness because of a dietary deficiency, a toxic relationship, or a broken spirit, and the present cause is addressed, that illness is cured. If we encounter another serious dietary deficiency, toxic relationship, or a broken spirit, we might acquire a new illness. It is not remission, and re-emergence of illness. It only appears so when we limit our view to by signs and symptoms. When viewed by cause, the cure is clear.

Alternative Cures

Does a homeopath, a naturopath, or a chiropractor, or a practitioner of Traditional Chinese Medicine, or Ayurveda, create more or fewer cures, than a conventional doctor?

These practitioners often use the same techniques as conventional doctors, recommending treatments for symptoms. We often see the word *works*. *"Which medicines, conventional or alternative works better?"* or *"Do alternative medicines work as well as conventional medicines?"* If it cures, there is no need for discussion. It's time to replace *works* with *cures*.

Debates, even clinical studies measuring differences between conventional and alternative medicines can often be summarized as a nonsense debate posing a nonsense question:

> *"Which treatment, conventional or alternative,
> does **not cure** better?"*

Cured is not defined for most diseases, not for conventional treatments, not for alternative treatments. When cured is not the goal, the treatment chosen makes little difference. For every alternative medicine in the alternative health store that doesn't cure, there is a conventional medicine in the pharmacy that doesn't cure either. If either could cure, the other would have no buyers. There would be no debate.

The strange truth about medicine today: most alternative medicines don't need to cure anything. They sell well because pharmaceutical medicines don't cure the same diseases. All sizzle, no steak. All bun, no beef. All smoke and no fire. All treatments and no cures.

Sometimes a naturopath, or a chiropractor, or another alternative practitioner, sometimes even a western medical doctor, spends more time with the patient, listens to the patient, talks to the patient, changes the patient and cures the illness. Not a zipless cure, because zipless cures are as rare as unicorns. A real cure that involves the patient, that emerges from changes in the actions and inactions of the patient. When a doctor, any type of doctor, or even a patient, without the aid of a doctor, aims for a cure, cures can be found.

But cures cannot be recognized. There are no statistics for cured. Cured is not defined. Cured cannot be proven, even when it is attained.

Invisible Cures

Cures are invisible. They cannot be tested scientifically. Conventional medicine ignores all cures. Cured is only defined when the cure is a medicine. Even those cures are ignored once they occur.

If you cure someone of a non-communicable disease, you are a Saint, or a miracle worker, not a doctor. If you claim to be able to cure, you're obviously insane, or perhaps just stupid, or a quack.

All cures are invisible today. It's impossible to prove their presence or absence. Even medicines designed to cure are currently marketed as treatments, not as cures.

Cure: *"Something that corrects or relieves a harmful or disturbing situation,"* **The American Heritage Dictionary of the English Language, Fourth Edition.**

Cure or Treatment?

Most medical treatments are *not cures*. *Working* without curing, without any design or intention to cure. If they cured, we could call them cures. News reporters, marketers, and sometimes even medical professionals often mistakenly refer to treatments as cures, especially in book titles and headlines, although less frequently in actual content.

Treatments that do not cure aim to minimize or limit the signs, symptoms, and damage of a disease. They can't address all signs and symptoms – and seldom remove any sign or symptom completely. Most treatments only work until the signs, symptoms, and damage grow in severity. Treatments can easily move the patient away from a cure while giving patients and doctor a false sense of improvement.

Signs and symptoms of illness are complex and varied, affecting body, mind, spirit, and community. Many treatment alternatives can claim to *work* with respect to signs and symptoms while making no attempt to address the cause, no attempt to cure. Of course, sometimes an illness is cured by natural healthiness, giving the impression that the treatment provided a cure.

Medical practitioners often refer to the standard of care as the best treatment. However, cures are not documented in any standard of care. The quality of a treatment depends on factors, that do not produce to cures. Every treatment that does not cure is an alternative treatment – that does not cure. All treatments have side effects, unintentional consequences. As treatments fails to cure in different ways the patient's natural healthiness and their illnesses respond in different ways.

Someday, perhaps, every *Standard of Care* will aim to cure.

There is seldom a best cure. Cures are sufficient, but not perfect.

Iatrogenic Illnesses

An iatrogenic illness is an illness caused by a treatment or a cure. There are many iatrogenic illnesses. Medicines and other treatments that do not cure that do not aim to cure, can cause iatrogenic illnesses, often euphemistically referred to as *side effects*. Cures, most notably transformation cures – but causal cures and injury cures as well, can also cause iatrogenic illnesses.

Conventional medicine notices iatrogenic illnesses as diseases when they are persistent, and often aims to prevent them. However, the concept of curing is rarely, if ever, applied to iatrogenic diseases. They might be cured by health – but not by medicines, because they were caused by medical treatments, that avenue is somehow closed off.

The curing of iatrogenic illnesses is no different from the curing of any other illness. Causal iatrogenic illnesses caused by persistent exposure to a toxic medicine are cured by addressing the iatrogenic process. Attribute illnesses caused by a treatment are cured with transformations. Iatrogenic injuries are cured with healing.

Curing Causal Illness

Cure: *(not defined)* Webster's Medical Dictionary, 3rd Edition
(not defined) The Oxford Concise Medical Dictionary, 9th Edition
(not defined) Barron's Dictionary of Medical Terms, 6th Edition

Many medical dictionaries do not contain an entry for cure. I have not seen a single dictionary definition of cure uses the word *cause*. Medicines cannot cure causal illnesses. We cure them with health.

A causal illness has a present process cause. It might be caused by an ongoing deficiency or excess of nutrients, or exercise, or other necessities and stresses of body, mind, spirits, community or environment. Because causal cure addresses a causal process, a cure for a causal illness is a process. A deficiency illness is cured by a process that addresses the deficiency on an ongoing basis. An illness caused by stress is cured by a process that addresses the stress on an ongoing basis.

Occasionally, a single cure or cure action can cure a causal illness. A repetitive stress illness might be cured with a new chair or a new job. In these cases, the cure re-defines the illness as caused by an attribute – the old chair, or old job. Hindsight might direct us to silly causes of illness, but no matter – as long as cures are found.

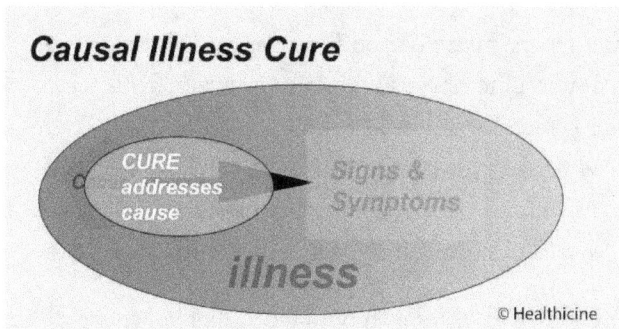

When the cause of an illness is addressed by a cure, the signs and symptoms fade, the illness fades, and healthiness grows. This might happen slowly or rapidly.

A causal illness element is cured when:

- The causal chain is successfully addressed on an ongoing basis,
- The signs and symptoms of illness are no longer present,
- Medicines to treat signs and symptoms, or to address the cause, are no longer needed.

A causal illness has a present cause and can only be cured by addressing the active present nature of the cause. Exploring a longer causal chain presents more opportunities to cure. When a causal chain splits into two or more independent chains, it presents two independent curable illnesses, such that addressing one chain provides only a partial cure.

On the other hand, when a curative action addresses several causal chains at once, it can re-define a compound illness into an illness element cured by a single action. An illness's complexity can sometimes be resolved by a successful cure or complexified by a partial cure.

When the illness is complex, multiple types of cure actions are necessary for a complete cure. When the causal illness causes injuries, healing cures are also required. When it caused negative attributes, transformational cures are required.

How Medicine Views Causal Illnesses

Conventional medicine treats many causal illnesses with little attention to cause. Conventional medicine has a single cure concept for infectious diseases – and no other concepts of cured for any causal illness. There is no medical test of cured for any non-infectious illness. Why? Because an illness with a cause is only cured by addressing the cause – and causes of non-infectious causal diseases are rarely be addressed with a medicine.

Conventional medicine views diseases as having complicated causes. The concept of an illness with a single cause and a causal chain does not exist for diseases. As a result, conventional medicine ignores many cures of simple diseases, and cannot see the possibilities for cures for complex or compound diseases.

Alternative medical practices offer little better for many reasons, perhaps most notably that conventional medicine holds the official definitions of medicines. When an alternative practitioner cures an illness, conventional medicine ignores the cure. Debates between conventional and alternative medical techniques are reduced to arguments about *not curative treatments*.

Anyone who claims to be able to cure any non-infectious disease is branded a quack, a fraud, a snake oil salesman. Conventional doctors intentionally avoid the word cure. Alternative medical practitioners have less fear of claiming cures and claiming the ability to cure. Their medical associations have less power over them.

Curing Injury Illness

Cure: *"Heal or make well"* Blakiston's,
"A healing or being healed" Webster's,
"The successful treatment of a disease or wound" Dorland's.

An illness is a hole in a healthiness. An injury illness is a hole in body, mind, spirit, or community. A severe stress might come from a process, or from an attribute that blocks a healthy process, causing an injury. An injury might come from internal causes; a stroke, a pulled muscle, or a hernia, or from external causes; from falling down the stairs, a car accident, a surgical procedure, or a gunshot. Injuries can also be caused by illness. Many treatments, including some cures, cause injuries.

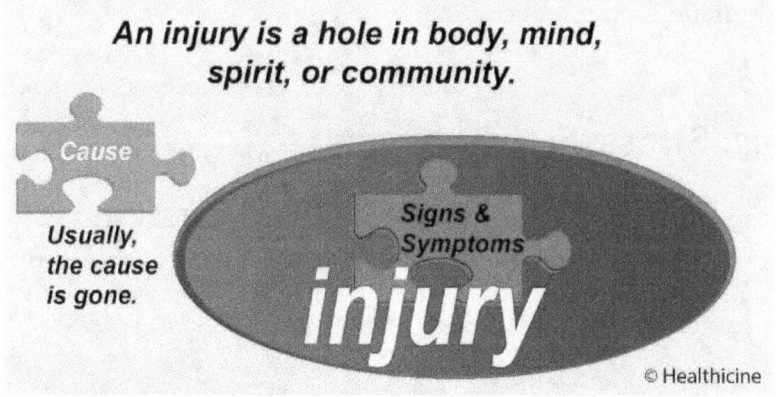

Injuries have signs and symptoms in the present and a cause in the past. The injury, the hole, causes the signs and symptoms of illness. The cause of the injury is in the past and cannot be cured.

Increscunt animi, virescit volnere virtus
(Spirits grow, and courage increases through wounds)
--- Friedrich Nietzsche

Every illness is a judgement. Every injury is a judgment. One person yells *"No Pain, No Gain!"* viewing injuries as a requirement for competition, necessary for improvement. Another might comment *"I was so stiff and sore it took me days to recover. I'll never do that again."* Some injuries, like arthritis injuries, can be caused by stress, or by lack of stress. *"Use it or lose it."*

Injuries come from severe forces or stresses. Sometimes a stress creates a causal illness. Sometimes it causes an injury. Sometimes it causes both a causal illness and an injury. An injury might be caused by a deficiency or an excess of: physical stress - in the body; mental stress - in the mind; emotional stress - of the mind and spirit; spirit stress – the stress of our intentions and goals; or a stress of community.

Signs and symptoms, the consequences of an injury, like the consequences of any illness extend throughout the entire hierarchy of diet, body, mind, spirits, and community.

Injuries: Stress vs Healthiness

When healthiness is lower, it's easier for a stress to create injuries. When healthiness is higher, it takes more stress to create an injury, and injuries are less severe.

Injuries Occur when Internal or External Stresses Overcome Healthiness and Strength

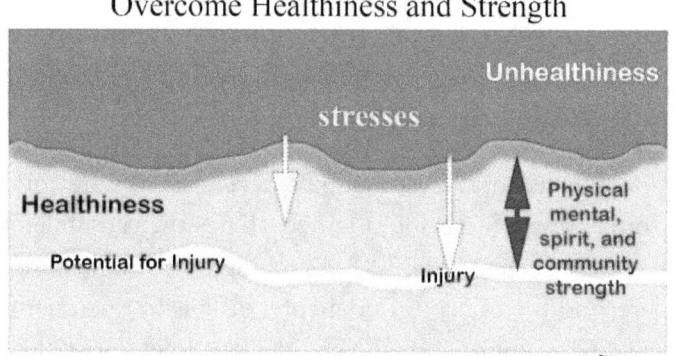

Strength exists separately from healthiness, although it is linked to healthiness. Too much strength can be unhealthy.

Like any cause of illness, an injury cause has a dual nature. An injury might occur when a stress is too severe for the body, mind, spirit, or community to tolerate. An injury might occur when a specific strength and healthiness of diet, body, mind, spirit, or community is so low that a normal or healthy stress causes an injury.

A single excessive stress might create several injuries. The concept of an injury illness element is not as critical to curing as with causal or attribute illnesses. The cause of the injury is gone. All injuries have the same cure: healing. We might consider a set of injuries, a result of a single cause to be an illness element, although several areas need to be healed. In other cases, it might be more effective to view a set of injuries with a single past cause as more than one illness.

Living entities take risks. We take risks with our body, and with our mind, our spirits, and our communities. It's a necessity of life. Risks sometimes lead to injuries. Life forms that avoid risk find fewer advantages, and are likely to be eaten, or out-competed by life forms that take risks more effectively. Gendered life forms have an advantage that the male, the more expendable gender, can take more risks and typically sustain more injuries. Females naturally take fewer risks. Their survival is more critical to the success of the species. Males can be more independent, and benefit from their independence, while females need more cooperative attributes, and benefit from those strengths. A gendered species can adjust and evolve faster with less danger to the entire species.

After a causal illness is cured, it is sometimes necessary to cure injury consequences. Conventional medicine often combines the causal illness and the injury illness into a single disease, searching for a single cure, a more complex cure, and then fails to find a cure, or fails to document a cure when it occurs. Conventional medicine does not track most cures, rarely documents cures for any disease, and does not have a useful concept of cured for injuries.

Healing

The natural healing force within each of us is the greatest force in getting well.
— Hippocrates

Injuries are cured by healing, by the natural, healthy processes of life.

The simplest living entity has injury repair mechanisms. Wounds are healed. When a cell with a wound on one side reproduces by division, one of the progeny might have no trace of the wound. The descendants of that cell are unharmed. The other cell line might further divide such that only one side has the injury. Over time, the injury can disappear as some of the cell lines die off. Tissues are self-repairing due to natural cellular replacement. Many injuries to organs and limbs can be repaired by health and healing.

Healing is independent of cause. It does not matter how an arm was broken, nor how the spirit was broken – healing proceeds based on the damage, and the healthiness of the patient, not on cause. Healing progresses independent of symptoms, independent of treatments, except treatments that aid healing.

Healing is also independent of the disease or the illness, except when a deficiency or excess of healing causes an illness.

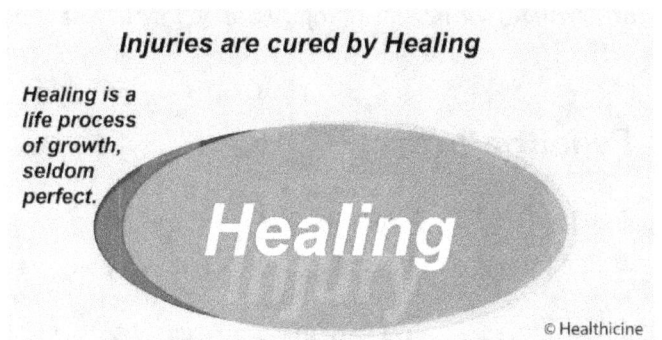

Healing masks over the injury, but the repair is seldom perfect.

Healing can only move forward, not backwards.

Perfection is impossible – cures do not require perfection to be judged cured. We might judge an injury to be cured when the wound has healed to a scar. At that point, we might view the scar as a negative attribute, but it is no longer the injury, no longer the injury illness. As a negative attribute it might, or might not, cause an attribute illness which can only be cured by transformation.

There are many ways to aid healing, to promote healing cures:

- improve the health of the patient,
- provide rest and resources that allow and assist healing,
- Stimulate healing processes, with physical, mental, spirit, and social exercise,
- nutrition,
- sometimes medicines to help the body to rest and recover.

Artificially increasing the rate of healing can result in problems that might be avoided by healing more slowly, at a more natural rate.

Injury Cured

An injury illness element is cured when:

- Healing is completed,
- signs and symptoms of the injury are gone,
- congestion is cleared, leakages have stopped,
- medicines for signs and symptoms of injury are no longer needed.

Injury Illness Proof of Cure

Conventional medicine does not judge injuries cured. Injuries are healed. The word cured is rarely, if ever used for injury illnesses.

Healing completed is a judgement. Judgements are necessary to cure injuries, to validate an injury cure.

How Medicine Views Injuries

> *The art of medicine consists of amusing the patient while nature cures the disease.*
> *-- Francois Marie Arouet Voltaire*

Conventional medicine performs best, not at healing injuries, but at addressing urgent, dangerous physical conditions. Emergency departments are the busiest place in any hospital or clinic. Conventional medicine excels at emergencies. But no emergency clinic can heal, healing comes from health. Patients are sent home to heal, to cure themselves. Of course, if a patient has many serious injuries, perhaps a burn patient, those will be attended to in detail. But once the patient is stable, they are often sent home to heal. Our bodies, minds, spirits, and communities can heal many injuries once immediate danger has passed. Little attention is paid to efficiency or effectiveness of healing.

Sometimes conventional medicine searches for medicines that boost healing unnaturally – and can be patented. Natural healing is ignored. There's no patent, no possibility of money or profit.

Although injury illnesses can occur in the body, the mind, the spirit, or the community of a life form, today's medical systems pay most attention to the body. Injuries to mind and spirits are often treated as injuries to the body, with drugs to suppress physical symptoms.

Conventional medicine often withholds treatments for illnesses, including injuries, because many medical treatments are dangerous and can cause injuries and even death. Even so, thousands of people die every year as a result of medicines, perhaps most by painkillers for what are seen as incurable injuries to body, mind, or spirit.

Healing is dependent on health. Many techniques that improve healthiness facilitate healing. Techniques to improve healthiness are not medicines. They are healthicines. Health is slow and steady. Healing takes time, and medical time costs money. It is more cost effective, in many cases, to send patients home to heal. Healing effectiveness is seldom measured.

When the patient has completed healing, there is seldom documentation of a cure. The follow-up, if any, is on the next regular medical checkup. If one patient heals faster, so much the better. If another patient heals slowly, a physician might note that the patient is healing slowly but rarely makes recommendations to optimize healing cures. Optimal healing is not important in a market-driven, product based, medical system. It produces fewer sales and less profit. Marketable medicines that produce faster healing can increase risk. There's little attention to the concept that healthier healing indicates a healthier patient. There are few, if any, studies of which injuries might benefit from slower healing vs others that benefit from faster healing. Sports doctors often aim for faster healing, even when it reduces overall healthiness. The goal is not health, it is to get a competitor back into the game.

When healing cures are aided by non-conventional medical techniques like chiropractic, Traditional Chinese Medicine, acupuncture, and others, conventional medicine often refuses to acknowledge any benefit.

Conventional medicine and alternative medicine often fail to study and understand differences between transformation and healing. Both study medical effects on signs and symptoms more than actual healing, actual curing.

Complex Injuries

Injuries can cause other illnesses. An injury can cause a change in habits, actions, or movements, resulting in more injuries. An injury might cause a change in diet, sometimes improving healthiness, sometimes leading to additional illnesses. An injury might block a natural flow, causing congestion, which might benefit healing with a scab, or block circulation and cause a failure of health and healing.

Causal or attribute illnesses can also cause injuries. A common cold might cause a nosebleed. Sometimes the illness that caused an injury is still present, causing more injuries. In this case, there are two elements of illness, the causal illness element and an injury illness element. Each needing to be cured.

Many illnesses can be cured before they can cause an injury. As a causal illness progresses uncured, it can cause more injuries, more serious injuries, until it is cured. Perhaps, as we study and practice cures, we cure more illnesses before injuries are caused. When an illness causes injury, we might view the injury as a failure to notice the illness, to address the cause with health, to cure before it causes injuries.

When the cause is still present, as in the next diagram, a complex illness exists, consisting of a causal illness element, and an injury illness element. An illness, with two elements of illness, requires two cures, one to address the cause, another to heal the injury.

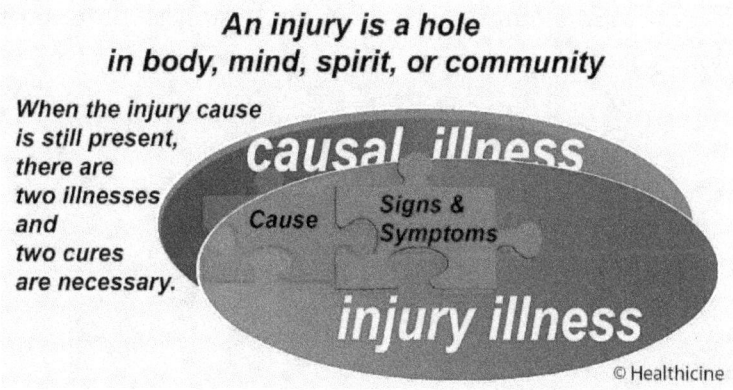

Because the causal illness persists, healing the injury illness only provides a partial, temporary cure.

Confusion between Healing and Transformation

Many books with the word cure in the title use the word healing in the contents, rarely using the word cure. Cure is an important marketing term, even as the basic concepts are ignored or misunderstood. Many of the cures presented or discussed are transformations. It's easy to be confused. Transformations cure attribute illnesses, but often cause injuries which require healing to complete the cure. Injuries are attribute illnesses – but not all attribute illnesses are injuries.

When we see references to cures that heal, if the author is using the word heal correctly, the illnesses being cured are injuries. However, medical professionals and writers often use the word heal for transformations. Transformations of cause are seldom recognized as cures. Alternative practitioners often refer to transformations of the patient – only the cause needs to be transformed.

Healing is a type of transformation, but not every transformation is a type of healing.

Every cure is a story, an anecdote. Health and healing are slow and steady. Healing cures seldom make interesting stories. Stories of transformations followed by healing are more interesting, get more press.

Curing Attribute Illness

Cure: *"To remedy or eradicate,"* Funk and Wagnalls Canadian College Dictionary, 1989.
"To remove or remedy something harmful or disturbing," The American Heritage Dictionary of the English Language, Fourth Edition

Most Attributes are Healthy

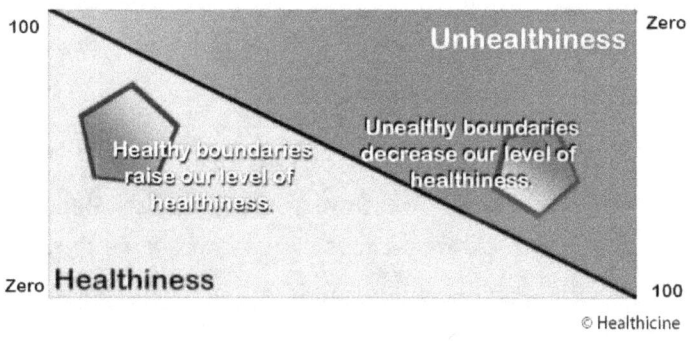

Life entities use attributes in the natural processes of living. Normally, they do not cause any illness. When an attribute causes a large drop in healthiness, illness can occur. We judge the attribute to be negative.

An attribute illness, like every illness, is a negative judgement. It exists when an illness or the signs and symptoms of illness are judged to be caused by a negative attribute. It can be difficult to determine if an attribute is truly positive or negative, healthy or unhealthy. A positive or neutral attribute might become negative over time, or in specific situations. This can happen at any level of diet, body, mind, spirit, or community.

In some cases, the judgement of a negative attribute is clear. In others, an attribute might be viewed beneficial by some, negative by others, or beneficial sometimes, negative at other times. Many attributes are negative in excess. Pessimism and optimism are attributes that can be healthy in moderation and unhealthy in excess.

Cause of a Negative Attribute

The cause of an attribute illness is the presence of a negative attribute. Every negative attribute has a cause because every cause has a cause. But the cause of an attribute is in the past. Finding and addressing causes of attribute illnesses can be useful to prevent future attribute illnesses – but seldom useful to cure. Negative attributes can be caused by faulty growth (cataracts, cleft lip, hernia, etc.), by injuries, or by faulty healing of injuries (callouses, scar tissue, relationship scars, or failures). They might be created by many internal or external forces.

We often think of illness as having an external cause, this valuable concept providing many cures. However, success with signs and symptoms by addressing an external cause can encourage us to ignore the poor health of the patient, possibly creating a chronic illness. Successfully treating the wrong cause fails to cure. Negative attributes often have causes external to the life entity, but the attribute, the cause of a present illness, is present, a part of the life entity, their community, or perhaps their environment.

Negative physical attributes might be caused by poor nutrition, exercise, or prior illnesses. Negative mind and spirit attributes can be caused by unhealthy mental processes, or unhealthy motivations or intentions. They might even be caused by success – when a success is linked to an unhealthy activity. Physical blockages of breathing or blood circulation can lead to death. In cases not so severe, they lead to illnesses like hypertension and Chronic Obstructive Pulmonary Disease (COPD). A physical, or body blockage might be scar tissue or other consequences of healing. Medical practice does not distinguish well between causes, or illnesses, of the mind, spirit, and community. Is PTSD a blockage of the mind, or the spirits of the afflicted? Are criminal activities, where the criminal is judged to be insane, a negative attribute of the brain, or the mind, or the spirits, or the community? The answers can only be provided by a successful cure. I am certain we can find examples of each. Conventional medicine treats physical, mental, and spirit illnesses with medicines – as if they are founded in the chemical composition of the body, and treats community attribute illnesses with prisons, as if the individual must be punished, not the community cured.

Curing attribute illnesses of mind, spirit, or community can require transformation of thoughts, perceptions, memories and beliefs. Negative community attributes might be caused by an individual or something in the community's past. A negative attribute might be a consequence of illness, of injury, of healing, of growth, or deterioration. It can also be caused by natural imperfections in, or natural consequences of the processes of life, living, and aging. But a past cause cannot be accessed to cure.

> *You don't fall ill, you slide. Sometimes very slowly, over a long period of abuse and lack of awareness.*
> *--- Thérèse Bertherat, Carol Bernstein*

Attribute causes often creep or slide into existence, growing slowly as time passes. They might be invisible until an illness progresses to a crisis, or until a person undertakes a new or infrequent activity. In these cases, an early diagnosis of cause, and a healthy cure, should be the goal.

Negative attributes can also cause injury. Acne blockages can cause infections. High blood pressure can lead to aneurysms, leakages. The presence of a physical scar can disrupt movement, resulting in accidents. Blockages and leakages of mind, spirits or community can result in severe illnesses, including mass murder – which our current systems treat as crimes, not symptoms of illnesses.

Attribute: Boundary Illnesses

The most common type of attribute illnesses are boundary illnesses. A boundary can be a fact, a physical, mental, spirit or community reality, often a real thing, sometimes an imaginary thing, a mindset, an attitude, or belief, separating inside from outside, often separating good from bad. Healthy living entities use boundaries to move forward. We build dams and bridges to move our society forward. Boundaries are a natural, healthy part of life and living. A boundary might be positive, or negative. If it's neutral, it's not a boundary.

The smallest life entity, a single cell, is defined by its cellular membrane separating inside from outside. If the cellular membrane becomes weak or unhealthy, the cell might die. Throughout its entire life, the cell must constantly maintain the health of the membrane.

A cell uses healthy boundaries to take in nutrients, excrete waste products, and block toxins from entry. As it succeeds, it grows and reproduces. When a boundary fails, the cell might die. A bodily tissue that forms a boundary for body parts has boundaries as well. Bodily organs have very clear boundaries, while organ system boundaries can be difficult to discern.

Humans have an organ, our skin, separating our body from the outside. The skin is a community of tissues, made up of many communities of cells, working in cooperation and competition. This membrane is essential to our healthiness. When it becomes too strong, too weak, or too unhealthy in many different ways, we too might suffer an illness, even die.

Humans have many physical, mental, spirit, and community boundaries which must be maintained, and sometimes destroyed, to maintain healthiness. Positive boundaries contribute to healthiness. Negative boundaries lead to unhealthiness and illness.

Boundaries can be things or processes. Every life entity, from a single cell to a community of humans, has and must maintain boundaries and boundary processes, to allow entry of positive health factors and exclude negative ones. These boundaries are never perfect. Life is about living, not about perfection.

Boundaries facilitate flows and blockages that are a necessary part of health. We often use boundaries as preventatives. Life forms also use boundaries to get things done. The stones across a stream are a boundary that helps us cross without getting our feet wet. Well-designed stairways are boundaries to help us climb with minimal risk. Boundaries might be physical, like skin, or a door, or mental, like attention and rules, emotional attributes like confidence and fear, or spirit attributes – like drive or boredom.

Positive boundaries help us to move forward and upwards, blocking out distractions. Negative boundaries can limit or disrupt healthy actions. Negative boundaries might block healthiness or leak healthiness.

Negative or unhealthy boundaries can cause attribute illnesses. A negative boundary might be a result of our imagination, of faulty beliefs, but the resulting illness is real, its effects are real, not imaginary. Good fences make good neighbors. Bad fences are a cause and a consequence of community illness. The bigger the physical, mental, spirit, or community wall, the more severe the illness that might result.

There are two main types of boundary failures, and two sides to each, any of which can lead to illness. Blockage might fail to allow the good to enter, or the bad to exit. Leakages allow negative factors to enter, or healthiness to drain from a life entity.

We're familiar with physical blockages. When someone moves their arm a certain way, their shoulder locks up. The other shoulder doesn't have this problem. Blockages can sometimes exist for long periods without being judged as an illness, sometimes without being noticed until we challenge ourselves in new ways. We compensate for blockages naturally, healthily. A mental blockage; "I don't like fish" might gradually cause a deficiency of nutrients likely to be found in fish, but not found in many other foods. Mental blockages can be transformed by understanding, or by correcting invalid perceptions or ideas. A spirit blockage diminishes intent, motivation, and passion, and can lead to feeling *"I'm bored,"* to depression, or even suicide. A community blockage, like a rule or law against a healthy activity, can lessen healthiness and create illness. Blockages can be caused by growth and healing. Healing, seldom perfect, often leaves blockages in body, mind, spirit, or communities.

Leakage attributes are another common cause of attribute illness, leaking healthiness or allowing unhealthiness to enter. Leakage attribute illnesses of the physical body include minor bruises and wounds, but most leakages are more subtle, ranging from faulty digestion and elimination of waste to leakage of attention and memories. Mental leakages can occur when we are distracted and forget what we need or need to attend. They can also occur when incorrect or negative facts intrude and become part of our belief systems, allowing truth to be mistaken or to leak out. It's not easy to be certain which facts, memories, calculations, or plans are correct. What was correct yesterday might not be correct today. When we become disoriented in our mental state, to the point where we cannot remember the day, or what to do in the morning, the afternoon, or the evening, we are suffering from a severe mental leakage, which might be an illness – or if incurable, a disability. Spirit leakage can create a leakage of motivation, intention, of faith in ourselves, or the entrance of motivations and intentions harmful to health, which can lead to illness.

Humans live in communities. We must continually create and maintain healthy boundaries in our communities. Leakage of self, in a community, can lead to one attribute illness; isolation to a different attribute illness, a blockage illness. The distinction between a blockage and a leakage depends on our perspective. We can always view a blockage as a failure to leak healthily, or a leakage as a failure of blockage.

Unhealthy boundaries have causes in the past. We cannot go back in time and address the cause. The present cause is not active. It's a thing not a process. Attributes cause illnesses by disrupting healthy life processes. Attribute illnesses must be cured by transformation, by changing the present attribute to a healthier state.

There are many different attribute illnesses and diverse types of transformational cures.

Blockage Illnesses

A negative blockage slows, blocks, or stops the healthy flows of a life entity

Our blood vessels provide a simple illustration of a blockage attribute illness. A blockage in a blood vessel might occur due to many causes, from external damage or pressure to internal growth, gradual deterioration, or other failure to facilitate a healthy flow.

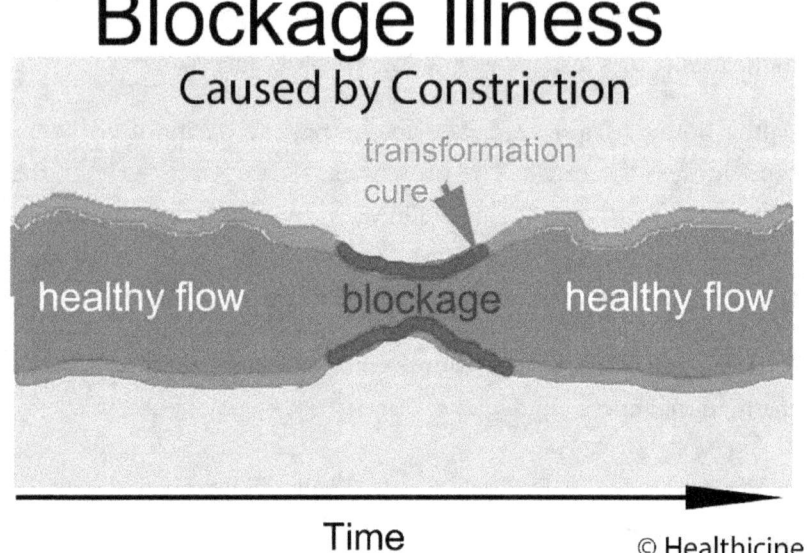

In the above image, a blockage slows or stops a natural flow of life and can result in congestion.

There are two basic ways for a blockage illness to be caused, by a constriction, or by an excessive flow.

High blood pressure is a common blockage caused by the inflexibility of veins and arteries. High blood pressure is a system-wide blockage of the circulatory system, which can have many consequences, causing many other illnesses.

A blockage might also be the result of increased or excessive flow which exceeds the natural ability of a life process.

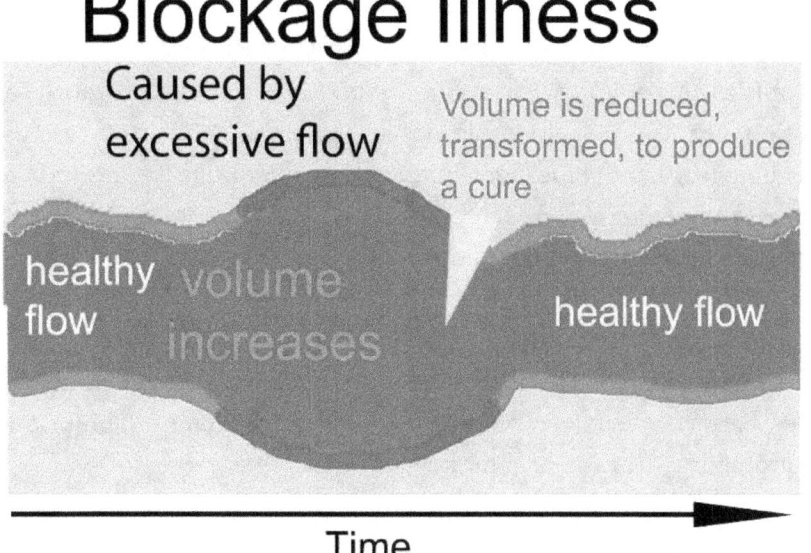

This graphic illustrates a blockage illness caused by an excessive flow as it arrives and as it is cured. A blockage attribute illness is cured by transforming the negative attribute. In the first case, the vessel needed to be transformed, in this case, the excessive flow is the cause that needs to be transformed.

Patients with high blood pressure might find their doctor giving two pieces of advice at once. Take ACE inhibitors, a medicine to loosen up blood vessels; and minimize salt consumption, in the belief that salt can increase the amount of fluid in the body, increasing blood pressure. Both treatments are symptomicines. They address the symptoms of the illness but do cure. The cure for a blockage is transformation. If the blood vessels are unhealthy, blocking healthy flows, the way to cure the illness is to health the blood vessels. Because the problem is system wide, it cannot be cured by surgery. It can only be cured by health. It might be more effective to view the progression of illness as causal, as caused by the patient's diet and exercise (or lack of exercise) activities and cured by addressing those causes. The cure proves the cause.

Blockages can occur in the physical body, like cataracts, or scar tissue, because of sudden or gradual injury. They can also occur in the mind, as simple as *"if you think you cannot, you are right."* In the spirits, the intentions or lack of intention in a depressed patient; or in the community, where blockages are often intentionally created to encourage conformity, or even as preventatives. Laws are community boundaries blocking specific actions – hopefully aiming for a healthy balance between the rights of individuals and those of communities. Laws can unhealthy for specific individuals or communities, and we need to constantly monitor and maintain legal boundaries to maintain healthy active balances between individual and community rights and responsibilities – for the health of it.

Leakage Illnesses

A leakage illness is a result of a weak or ineffective boundary. Life boundaries need to be permeable, to let good things (nutrients, good thoughts, healthy motivating spirits, good friends and companions) enter our lives, and impermeable to keep out bad things (poisons, toxic thoughts, demotivators, and enemies). They must be permeable, to let bad things out, and impermeable to keep good things from leaving. We maintain life boundaries at every level, body, mind, spirit and community. Physical boundaries exist and must be maintained at cellular levels, at tissue levels, at organ and organ system levels, and for the entire body. An unhealthy boundary might leak unhealthiness out of body, mind, spirits, and communities or allow unhealthiness to leak into body, mind, spirits, and communities.

Like a blockage illness, a leakage illness is cured by transforming the attribute to healthiness. In many leakage injury illnesses, the curative transformation can only accomplished naturally by health or healing.

Blockage and leakage illnesses often occur together. A blockage can cause a rupture, leading to a leakage. A leakage can cause an accumulation that creates a blockage. Illness uncured can cause illness.

Transformation: Curing Attribute Illnesses

Attribute illnesses are cured by transforming: releasing, repairing, removing, or changing the negative attribute. The term used in this text is transformation. Transformations health negative attributes. Once a negative attribute is transformed to be neutral or even positive, two additional processes may be necessary; clearing congestion, and healing damage caused by the illness and the transformation.

There are many types of transformation. Curative transformations might occur in the body, the mind, the spirits, and the communities – depending on the negative attribute. Bandages might block physical leakages while they are transformed by healing. Leakages of body, mind, spirits, and community healthinesses are cured by many different types of transformations, and each attribute cause might have many potential curative transformations.

When the cause of an illness is a negative attribute, the cure is transformation and healing. Addressing leakage and congestion are important but do not cure.

Other Attribute Illnesses

Any illness cured by a transformation can be viewed as an attribute illness. Dentists transform teeth; priests transform spirits; counsellors transform relationships. Many illnesses which cannot be cured by simple healing; and cannot be cured by addressing the cause, can be cured by transformation of the present cause.

Attribute Illness Cured

An attribute illness of body, mind, spirit, or community is cured by transformation of the present cause to a neutral or healthy state. Sometimes they can be cured by transformations that allow the entity to live with the attribute without illness, like eyeglasses that transform vision. Transformation of a negative attribute often results in injuries which require healing to complete the cure.

An attribute illness element is cured when:

- The negative attribute has been transformed to a non-negative state,
- Healing of injuries caused by the transformation has completed,
- The signs and symptoms of the illness are no longer present,
- Medicines for signs and symptoms are no longer needed.

Attribute Illness Proof of Cure

Conventional medicine has no general concept of an attribute illness. Cured is not defined for any attribute illnesses except when the attribute is an infection cured by surgery. In reality, surgery is often an attribute cure. Ranging from minor, like extracting a sliver or an ingrown toenail, to complex procedures like a heart transplant. But today's conventional medicine has no definition and sees no proof of cured.

How can we be certain an attribute illness is cured? Often, when an attribute is changed, we cannot go back to the previous state. We cannot undo a surgery to test if it was the cure. Sometimes, we can reverse the attribute change to see if a new illness occurs. If we cured myopia with glasses, we can easily remove the glasses and see the illness again, because the eyes were not actually transformed. However, if we cure myopia with eye exercises – proof of cure is much more difficult. Every cure is an individual case, an anecdote, insufficient for bureaucratic proof.

Some negative attributes are attributes of the mind, the spirit, or the community which can be changed. An illness caused by a negative attribute of mind or spirit might be cured by transformation of belief or intention. A patient might consult a doctor about a worrisome illness, a new bump or blemish on their skin – and the doctor might simply explain it to be a mole or other natural feature, curing the illness with community knowledge. When a patient *sees the light* and understands the perceived attribute and illness as normal, even healthy, an illness has been cured. The belief that cures only come from medicines limits our understanding, limits our successes.

Enlightenment is a form of transformation, a form of cured. We might view a person desperately seeking enlightenment as having an illness of spirit, which is cured when enlightenment transforms their mind and spirits. The cure might also lead to a transformation of their body, mind, and their communities.

Transformation is also a powerful preventative. Adolescents are in a transitional state between being children and adults, a natural transformation. Sometimes they get stuck or are held back in their development. Many societies and many communities have transformation rituals that signify adulthood to the individual and to the community. Many people in South America celebrate quinceañera, the transition from childhood to womanhood at 15. Jewish children celebrate Bar Mitzvah, signifying the age at which they become responsible for their actions. High school students and gangs often have initiation ceremonies or requirements before a new person can enter the community. These transformations have two sides because they are about community. The community recognizes that the person has attained the status of a member, and the individual sees this recognition as defining and transforming themselves. In some cases, the transformation might be slight – when the child already has the attributes of an adult, in others, it might be dramatic, preventing many problems even curing illnesses. Boundaries between the individual and the community are weakened in some ways, such that the individual is a member, and strengthened in other ways, by having the individual as a new member. Anyone who cannot pass the initiation might be seen as an outsider, as weak or sick. Of course a transformation to enter a negative community, like a gang might cause illnesses.

How Medicine Views Attribute Illnesses

Attribute and boundary illnesses are phrases not commonly discussed in medical texts. However, many common medical terms describe blockages which might occur due to illness or injury: arrest, clogging, congestion, difficulty, obstruction, barrier, hindrance, impediment, resistance, stoppage, and others that refer to unhealthy leakage: hernia, aneurysm, bleeding, blisters, and runny nose. There are indirect references to blockages and congestion found in many dictionary definitions of cure. The American Heritage Dictionary of the English Language, Fourth Edition defines cure as *"4. To remove or remedy something harmful or disturbing: cure an evil."* Merriam-Webster's College Dictionary 11th Edition, 2003 suggests, *"To restore to health, soundness or normality,"* which might apply to any illness, and clearly to attribute illnesses.

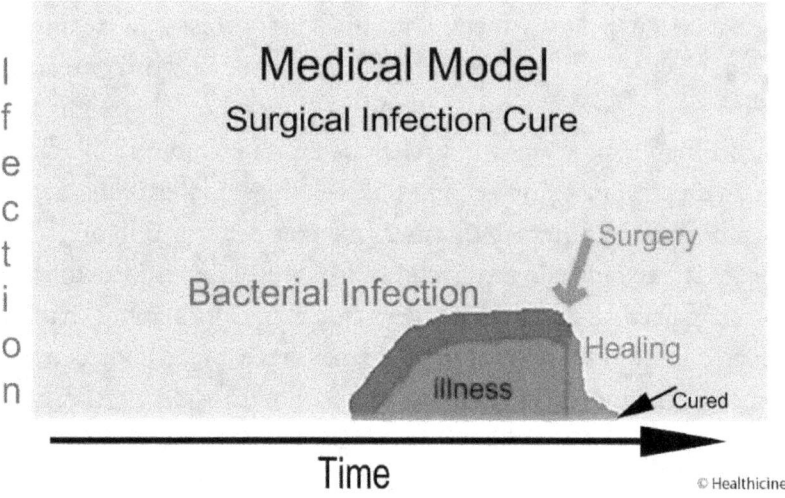

Surgery is a type of transformation. We have seen this image before, which shows a cure by transformation, followed by healing. Surgical cure of an infection is recognized as a conventional medical cure. An antibiotic might cure by addressing the infection cause and letting the body heal. Some infections cannot be cured with antibiotics, only by surgery, so we view the infection as a negative attribute, cured by surgical transformation.

Conventional medicine often uses transformational techniques in physiotherapy, but seldom uses the word cure. Physiotherapy that cures can easily be ignored – the patient, or their illness, disappear from the system. Slow transformations are more difficult to document as cures. Patients with more complex conditions often have some disability aspects that can be treated, but not cured. Those that can be cured might take long periods of time, giving the impression that physiotherapy and similar transformational treatments like massage, and chiropractic, cannot cure. When we expect only perfect cures, we fail to see many cures.

Alternative medical practitioners often misunderstand the concepts of attribute illnesses, confusing transformation and healing, even as they cure. An osteopath, a chiropractor or a massage therapist might unblock a muscle, tendon, an area of the fascia, or a joint to produce a transformation cure. Note: many chiropractic and massage treatments do not aim to cure. An osteopath might rarely use the word cure, even as they cure. The word cure is forbidden. A psychologist might help transform a mental blockage, or a relationship - a community blockage. A parent, a mentor, or a priest might unblock the spirit, enabling natural healing processes to complete a cure. But they are not doctors – and cures are not recognized. Even cures brought about by doctors are seldom recognized as cures. Forgiveness is a transformation; that can sometimes cure an illness of spirit that may have existed for decades. Sometimes a random event, like a whack on the side of the head, transforms a perspective, curing an illness of the mind or spirit. A hypnotist might cure by creating a healthy blockage (enabling a person to stop smoking) or by repairing a leaking mental or spirit boundary. A comedian might cure illnesses, by releasing the tension of a negative boundary, or by opening a patient's awareness. Many doctors deliberately use humor in their practice. Norman Cousins in the book, *"Anatomy of an Illness as Perceived by the Patient"* describes the active use of laughing to aid his cures; after doctors gave up on his incurable condition which could not be diagnosed as a disease.

Cured is not medically defined when accomplished by most transformations. Cured is not defined for attribute illnesses except when the attribute is an infection cured by surgery. Surgery is often an attribute cure.

A psychologist, friend, parent, priest, mentor or even an enemy might provide surgical transformation of mind, of memories and beliefs, or spirits, the motivations and intentions, or of community, of relationships between people. But conventional medicine does not recognize these actions as curing and does not recognize these results as cures, even when a disease disappears. Conventional medicine, blind to cures, can only see remission.

Attribute clearing techniques like surgery and leakage repair techniques like stitches and bandages can also be useful in curing injuries, helping them to heal.

The current practice of medicine does not see the concept of an attribute as a cause and type of illness, although such diseases are recognized.

Attribute Illness, Injury, or Disability?

The distinction between an injury and an attribute illness can be difficult to discern. There is, in theory, a simple technique. To cure an attribute illness the negative attribute must be transformed. If it can be healed, it is an injury illness – healing is also a transformation. Sometimes the distinction is determined by the success of a cure.

If it is cured by a transformation, it was an attribute illness. After transformation, an attribute cure often requires a healing cure, because transformations can create injuries.

Maybe you've noticed an overlap between an injury and a leakage boundary illness? Both might be viewed as a hole in the body.

Three Elements of Illness

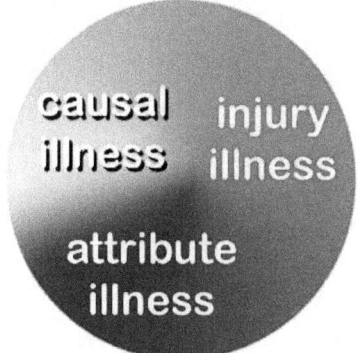

When we look at any element of illness, we will always find gradations and overlap between causal illness elements, injury illness elements, and attribute illness elements. How can we be certain which classification is correct? Only by curing.

When addressing a present process cures, it was a causal illness. When making the patient's life processes healthier cures the illness, a healthy cure, it was a causal illness – caused by the patient's lack of healthiness. When healing cures, it was an injury illness. When transformational cures succeed, it was an attribute illness.

Every illness is a judgement. An attribute illness, a handicap, and a disability have similar features. Handicaps and disabilities often entail stigmas outside of the issue of cure – beyond the scope of this book. By definition, every curable illness has the potential to be cured.

If a disability is cured, it was an attribute illness. If it is healed, it was an injury illness. If it disappears? We're not certain, but it was probably an injury. Health is slow. Sometimes healing takes a long time. When an attribute illness is judged to be incurable, it is judged to be a disability, a handicap, or perhaps simply a natural feature.

Cures are defined by success. Success is defined by cures. Treatments that do not cure can sometimes move our perception around the circle, pointing to other ways to cure, but only when we aim to cure.

Curing Chronic Illness

There are three basic elements of illness, causal illness elements, injury illness elements, and attribute illness elements, each having a unique type of cure, respectively: a causal cure, a healing cure, and a transformational cure.

Each type of illness can also be a chronic illness when the cause has a chronic attribute. A chronic bacterial infection is a chronic infection illness with a chronic cause. Chronic injury illnesses have chronic stress causes. Attribute illnesses are chronic by nature until their causes are transformed, unless they are caused by temporary attributes.

We can view the cause of the chronic nature of an illness as a higher-level cause. When a cause repeats or persists over time, the persistently present nature of the cause is a chronic cause, that creates a chronic illness. In many cases, a single occurrence of a process or injury cause is not sufficient to cause illness. Chronic illness only emerges, by definition, after an extended period, as the problem builds. Obesity is a chronic illness, but the cause, eating, does not cause obesity until it becomes chronic. People who are obese are told to go on a diet. A diet cannot cure a chronic disease unless it transforms the chronic nature of the cause.

Sometimes the chronic attribute of the illness is a habit, which can be changed or replaced with a healthier habit to bring about a cure.

When a stress is chronic, it creates a chronic illness. (Note: this is not the illness often referred to as *stress* which will be discussed later under the name stress-stress.) In many cases, a stress that causes a chronic stress illness is healthy when not chronic.

Repetitive stress injuries are chronic illnesses, caused by a chronic stress. Conventional medicine does not recognize chronic causes of mind or spirits. Such illnesses are always attributed to physical causes.

Chronic bacterial infections are chronic illnesses caused, not by bacteria, but by either the chronic presence of dangerous bacteria or the presence of a chronic level of unhealthiness that allows even healthy bacteria to invade and create infections. Chronic dietary deficiencies can cause chronic mental or spirit illnesses, which can cause further illness. In each case, the cure is to address not the cause, but the chronic nature, the chronic attribute of the cause.

Chronic illnesses are cured with health, by improving the health of the patient, their diet, bodies, minds, spirits, communities or environment. Health is every day, slow and steady. Regaining and maintaining health is slow and steady. Cures, as well, are often slow and steady.

Medical treatments sometimes cure chronic attribute illnesses by transforming the cause, but cannot cure chronic causal illnesses nor chronic injury illnesses.

Curing Chronic Causal Illnesses

Addressing the chronic attribute of a chronic illness requires identification of a chronic cause, an understanding of why the cause is chronic. Chronic diseases often require multiple cures, because they easily accumulate causes and thus consist of multiple elementary chronic illnesses.

Sometimes the chronic illness appears to be an episodic illness, caused by an unhealthy trigger. Some triggered illnesses can be deflected when the patient learns to recognize and disarm trigger events. However, triggered illnesses consist of the pressure of an unhealthiness just below the threshold of illness. If the cause of the unhealthiness is addressed, the danger of the trigger is removed. If not addressed, another trigger can emerge, releasing the unhealthy pressure as an illness. Often as the pressure is released, the unhealthiness that has accumulated is released and fades.

Most chronic illnesses rise and fall continually in cycles, even as they progress negatively, or towards a cure. Chronic illnesses sometimes disappear mysteriously, when the health of the patient or the environment changes, without conscious intention of doctor or patient. These cures are easily ignored, or dismissed, a cure, requires no attention. They are often dismissed as placebo effects by medical professionals and others. There are no placebo cures. Every cure has a real cause.

Curing Chronic Injuries

When the cause of an injury is persistent, there exists a chronic injury illness. Each individual presence of cause creates a minor injury, often not at the level of an illness. The sequence of injuries is a meta-cause, creating a chronic illness. These illnesses are sometimes called repetitive stress injuries, repetitive strain injuries, or work-related disorders.

A secretary might develop carpal tunnel syndrome from excessive stress, or bad posture. The cure is to address the chronic cause Attempts to cure the illness without addressing the chronic cause are doomed to fail.

There are also chronic injuries to mind, spirits, and communities. However, these are not recognized as types of disease – all diseases are designated as physical as if only the body can be injured.

Curing Chronic Attribute Illnesses

Attribute illnesses are naturally chronic. They persist until the attribute causing the illness is transformed or removed. If the transformation or removal caused injuries, those are another cure element which must be healed.

Stress, Chronic Stress and Stress-Stress

We can view every illness as caused by a stress and cured by addressing the stress. A chronic illness is caused by a chronic stress, one that persists over time.

Often when we think of illness caused by stress, we refer to *mental stress,* the stress of having and attending to many stresses at one time. Multiple chronic stresses can collect in body, mind, spirit, and communities. They can disrupt the mind and depress the spirits.

> *"The number one root of all illness, as we know, is stress." – Marianne Williamson*

> *"What you focus on grows, what you think about expands, and what you dwell upon determines your destiny." Robin S. Sharma*

Many stresses of body, mind, spirits, and community have a nature similar to pain. When we focus on our pain, we can magnify it such that it becomes unbearable. Stress is magnified by attention, magnified by anxiety. We sometimes dismiss stress by paying no mind. This might be a useful or an incorrect action depending on the situation.

Stress-stress, stressing about stress, is learned. We can learn to magnify our stress-stress, without realizing we are doing so. Stress can also be taught. Marketers sell anxiety: are your teeth whiter than white? do you need X? ask your doctor about Y? Marketers want us to buy things. When we are stressed, we are more likely to buy things to relieve our stress. News reporters want us to listen to and read their stories, so news stories are written to stress our emotions, deliberately raising stress. Television drama and advertising are designed to manipulate our emotions, to create stress, to keep us watching. Tension, stress, is deliberately increased before the commercials. Commercials often contain humor and are designed to increase *buy-stress*. Humor often creates the impression that buying will reduce stress.

Life makes healthy use of stress, and as a result, stresses can easily accumulate. Accumulated stress can create compound illnesses requiring more than one cure. It can also create chronic illnesses caused by the stress of stress.

We can also learn techniques to minimize stress-stress, to cure illnesses caused by stress-stress. Focussing on simple tasks like breathing, chopping wood, or other activities reduces stress, by taking our attention away from it. Stress, like pain, can be real, or imaginary, and it can be difficult to determine which is which.

One important technique for addressing illnesses caused by stress-stress is to do with being in the *present*. Stress-stress blurs our attention, constantly looking to the past with regret *"I should have done X,"* or to the future with fear *"What if...?"* When we attend to the present, many stresses fall away. Meditation, yoga, Tai Chi, even simple exercise like a daily walk, can bring our attention back to the present and help us find many cures.

Stress illnesses are rarely treated with intention to cure. Cured is not defined for any illness caused by stress on the mind, the spirit, or the community. Instead, we buy medicines that diminish symptoms and suck it up as the levels of stress rise higher and higher.

Chronic Illness Cured

A chronic illness element is cured when:

- The chronic attribute of the cause has been addressed,
- If an underlying illness is the cause, it is also cured,
- Healing is completed,
- Signs and symptoms are no longer present,
- Medicines to treat the signs and symptoms of the illness are no longer needed.

Chronic Illness Proof of Cure

Conventional medicine currently views chronic illnesses as incurable and has little interest in studying cures when they occur. In conventional medicine, there is no proof of cured for any chronic illness.

Chronic illnesses are attribute illnesses, a result of the chronic attribute of the cause. Often a chronic illness presents two illnesses that must be cured, one a direct result of the cause and another a result of the chronic nature of the cause.

We cannot prove that obesity is cured by over-eating to see if it returns. It will only return as a result of chronic eating. On the other hand, a return to chronic over-eating will bring signs and symptoms of additional weight, well before obesity occurs again. Many chronic illnesses creep slowly and provide ample evidence to understand cured.

When a chronic illness is cured by adding something, we can often test the cure by removing the new attribute. If chronic conditions were cured by adding a habit, like a daily walk or a resolution to maintain a positive attitude, we can easily reverse the new attribute to see the effect. If the illness returns, we prove the cure by its absence.

In some cases, there is danger in testing the cure. Many chronic illnesses create disabilities – and testing the cure risks additional disability which cannot be cured.

How Medicine Views Chronic Illness

Conventional medicine has no comprehension of the fact that a chronic illness always has a chronic cause. Chronic illnesses are viewed as mysterious, incurable diseases, which must be accepted. The common recommendation has become a mantra of conventional medicine, to *"learn to live with"* the disease.

It's easy to understand. No medicine can address the *chronic attribute* of a cause. No medical treatment can cure a chronic disease – unless it cures by transformation. No medicine can address a chronic cause unless the cause is a physical attribute.

Alternative medical practitioners often cure chronic diseases, by spending more time with individual patients, helping the patient to see, and address the chronic attribute of the cause. But alternative practitioners accomplish this without a comprehensive theory of chronic disease – and their successes are not recognized by conventional medicine. Conventional medicine holds the (non-)definition of cure and cured is not defined for chronic diseases. All cures are ignored. Chronic diseases cured by conversation, by hypnotism, or by illumination or enlightenment cannot be evaluated. Cured is simply not defined.

When a patient cures a chronic disease by changing their habits, an individual doctor might recognize the cure, but the medical systems do not track cures. Every cure is an anecdote. Every cure of a chronic disease is just another anecdote. Even a cure encountered in a clinical study is an anecdote, which can only be ignored when cured is not defined in the parameters of the study.

How to Cure A Chronic Illness

Norman Cousins' famous book **Anatomy of an Illness as Perceived by the Patient** is the story of a complex cure, requiring many cure elements. Many doctors find it a fascinating book. I suspect part of the fascination is the mysterious nature of the cure – which is not resolved in the book.

It is important to note that Cousins had a serious illness, but not a disease. He reports that his doctor *"reviewed the reports of many specialists he had called in as consultants. He said there was no agreement on a precise diagnosis."* His condition was serious – one specialist advised that he had one in 500 chance of surviving, that he had never witnessed a recovery from this comprehensive condition.

Perhaps if Cousins had received a diagnosis of a disease, it would also have come with a prognosis and a *recommended treatment that does not cure*, with advice that he *learn to live with* his disease. Cousins might have never cured his illness, might have never written the book.

How did Cousins cure his illness, when the many doctors he consulted could not offer useful advice, much less a cure?

Norman Cousins believed in himself. He quotes Dr. Schweitzer, *"The witch doctor succeeds for the same reason all the rest of us succeed. Each patient carries his own doctor inside him."* Cousins consulted many doctors. When none offered a cure, he set out on his own.

Cousins' actions did not tackle the illness directly. Instead, he worked steadily to improve his health, healthiness, and healing. One of the most effective techniques to cure any illness is to improve healthiness in as many ways as possible, sometimes over a long period of time.

Cousins took massive doses of Vitamin C – not as a medicine – as an aid to healing the damage done by the illness, long before Pauling recommended it. He avoided drugs for symptoms, and comments, *"many people tend to regard drugs as though they were automobiles. Each year has to have its new models, and the more powerful the better."*

Cousins advises – and spends an entire chapter on pain, titled *"Pain is Not the Enemy."* Cousin's learned to laugh with his illness and believes this was a fundamental component of his cure.

Cousins does not use the word cure – I suspect if he had, many doctors would have dismissed his story outright. He says, *"Is the recovery a total one? Year by year, the mobility has improved. I have become pain-free, except for one shoulder and my knees, although I have been able to discard the metal braces."* And *"I was sufficiently recovered to go back to my job at the Saturday Review full time again, and this was miracle enough for me."*

Cures are forbidden. More forbidden for chronic diseases. Impossible for chronic illnesses that cannot be diagnosed as a disease. Remission or recovery is are acceptable claims because they require little proof other than diminished signs and symptoms. When every cure requires perfection, every claim becomes a miracle.

How Cesar Millan Cures Chronic Illness

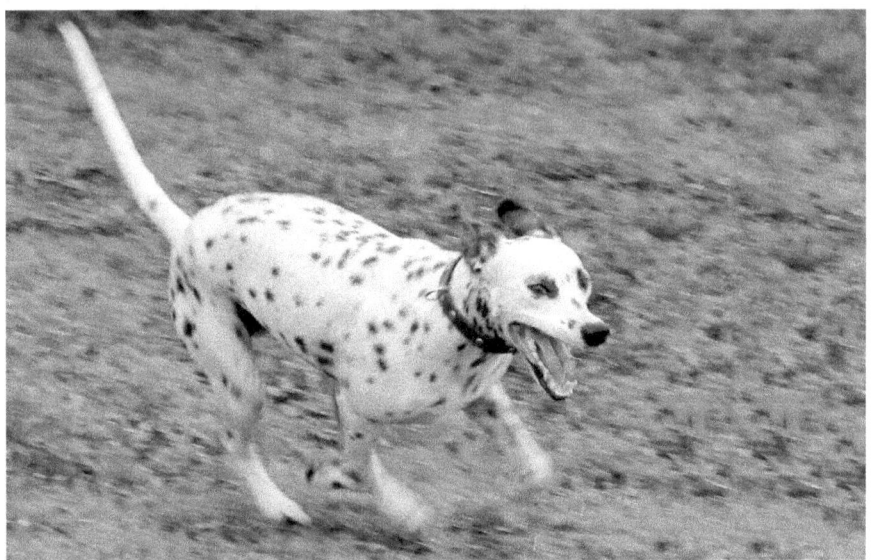

The Center for Managing Chronic Disease advises, *"Chronic Disease is a long-lasting condition that can be controlled but not cured."* They are simply wrong. What they should have said is:

Medicines cannot cure chronic diseases.

Let's take a walk with Cesar Millan, the dog whisperer.

If you've seen Cesar's popular television show, you will recognize the themes, but you might be surprised to learn how Cesar cures.

Many people with a chronic dog problem first contact Cesar by telephone. We know it's a chronic problem – or they would have already fixed it. Cesar only gets chronic dog problems. They talk to Cesar, and he listens. Cesar doesn't talk or listen to the dog. There is no need. Then Cesar comes to visit. What happens next?

When Cesar comes to visit, he doesn't visit the dog. In many cases, he hardly acknowledges the dog when he enters the house. Cesar greets the owner, talks and listens to the owners. He is aware of the dog, noticing the dog and dog's behavior, but not attending to it. Sometimes, especially with a dog displaying a lot of symptoms, Cesar will make a point of establishing his dominance, but he does not speak to the dog in human language, nor by barking at the dog.

Cesar looks at and listens to the owner. This is where he finds the cause of the disease. The dog has all the symptoms, but the owner has the present cause. The present cause is key to the cure.

Cesar creates a prescription for the dog owner. Not a medicine. Medicine cannot cure chronic illness. If we medicate the dog, it will be less of a dog. When the medication wears off, it might be less controllable. The prescription needed is action and activity. Action and activity for the dog. But the real, effective cures are actions and activities for the owner. The owner has the problem, not the dog.

The prescription might be unique for each owner, but the goals are clear – to make the owner a healthy owner and in doing so, to make the dog a healthy dog. To health the relationship between the dog and the owner. Cesar doesn't medicate the dog, nor the owner, he cures with health.

One of Cesar's first goals is to give the owner a sense of control. When Cesar mock bites the dog, he's not teaching the dog. The dog understands without a lesson. Cesar is teaching the owner that the dog is a dog, teaching the owner that healthy actions lead to healthy dog behavior. When the owner sees Cesar interact with the dog, they begin to see the source of the problem. When someone complains of a problem dog, the dog is rarely the problem. The dog is a dog. The problem is chronic. It persists over time. The cause of the illness is not in the dog, it's in the owner, in the relationship between the dog and the owner. Cesar provides a prescription for the relationship. But, Cesar can only make recommendations to the owner. The dog doesn't listen to Cesar, much less remember what Cesar says.

Cesar prescribes specific activities for the owner - with the dog, of course, designed to make the dog, and the owner, and their relationship, healthier. Cesar healths communities of dog and owner.

Cesar prescribes specific activities based on the active cause, not the symptoms. The owner can make changes. The dog will change when the owner changes. In many cases, the owner successfully carries out the activities designed to change their habits with regards to the dog, and the chronic illness goes away. Unhealthy habits are replaced with healthy habits. It might take two or more stages, due to complexity. Sometimes because the owner has difficulty changing. Perhaps the prescription was too strong and a slower, more gradual change is required, or perhaps a different prescription. But there is never a prescription for the dog - only for the Alpha Dog, the owner.

Many dog problems are boundary illnesses, cured by healthing boundaries. Perhaps the dog is too territorial, defending imaginary boundaries too strongly. Perhaps it is too timid, relying entirely on the owner to define boundaries, leaking confidence. Cesar transforms the relationship, such that the unhealthy boundaries become healthy, the invisible cause of illness disappears, and the illness fades.

The prescribed activities transform the relationship between the dog and the owner into a healthy relationship, and the dog is cured.

Does Cesar ever fail? Does he ever meet a chronic dog illness he cannot health? Yes, it does happen sometimes. Sometimes the specific community, the relationship between owner and dog, and perhaps other family members, cannot be healthed. Sometimes a dog has been so injured by past relationships with people, that it has acquired negative attributes preventing the relationship from being healthed. Sometimes the owner cannot change. In these situations, for the health and safety of all parties - separation is the only solution. Separation is sometimes a necessary step toward curing an unhealthy relationship. Sometimes a permanent separation is required.

What has this to do with chronic diseases in people? Chronic diseases cannot be cured by medicine. But chronic disease, in many cases, can be healthed - if the damage has not gone too far. Even when there is serious damage, healthing the situation often stops and can reverse the progression of the illness.

There is no Cesar Millan for chronic disease in people. There is no Cesar, who can ignore the dog, ignore the disease, and health the patient, or more to the point - teach the patient to health themselves. Medical doctors are not trained to separate causes of chronic illness in a patient's body, mind, spirit, and community from symptoms of the body, mind, spirit, and communities of the patient. Current disease names illustrate this confusion. Is heart disease an attribute disease of the heart, only cured by surgical transformation, or is it caused by poor diet and exercise, cured by healthing those processes. The name *heart disease* is used for both conditions. But there is no cure for heart disease. It's easier to treat the body with a surgery, or a medicine to address symptoms, and ignore cause, ignore cures.

Our medical systems consistently make several errors with chronic illness:

- failure to understand that chronic diseases have chronic causes
- medicating and managing the symptoms
- not looking for present process or attribute causes
- no intention to cure, assuming there is no cure, that a cure is not possible
- not recognizing, not studying cures even when they occur.

Chronic illnesses have chronic causes. Conventional medicine views an illness as chronic if it lasts three months or more. This artificial distinction is only necessary when the cause is not known. When the cause of an illness is understood, the illness can be judged chronic or not chronic, by studying the cause. If the cause is chronic, if the cause persists over time, the illness is chronic.

Injuries cannot be chronic, because the cause of the injury is gone. A chronic repetitive stress illness, often called a chronic injury, always has a chronically present process or attribute cause.

Chronic negative processes can cause chronic illnesses. Curing a case of an infection, or a dietary deficiency does not cure when the cause and the illness are chronic. It is necessary to find and address the chronic attribute of the cause. A chronic infection has a cause and a chronic cause. A chronic dietary deficiency has a cause, and a chronic cause. When a chronic illness exists for a long time, there are often more than two causes, and therefore more than two cures necessary, because chronic conditions accumulate causes. Sometimes a chronic process changes before the arbitrary three-month period passes – and the medical system fails to recognize the illnesses as chronic. It also fails to recognize the cure.

The other cause of a chronic illness is a negative attribute. Damage to the body that cannot be healed might be a chronic physical cause of illness. Negative attributes of mind, like incorrect information or memories, can cause chronic actions leading to chronic illness. Attribute causes can exist in diet, body, mind, spirit, community or environment. They exist until they are transformed. Sometimes an attribute is transformed before the arbitrary three-month period passes and we might judge them temporary, not chronic.

Many chronic attribute illnesses grow more severe over time because the negative attributes are caused by a negative process. Glaucoma, diabetes, heart disease are complex illnesses with chronic causes leading to chronic consequences that cannot be healed, to damage that cannot be healed but might be transformed.

Some of the chronic diseases identified by the Center for Managing Chronic Disease include allergy, Alzheimer's, asthma, breast cancer, diabetes, epilepsy, glaucoma, heart disease, and obesity. The very name of the organization, "Center for Managing Chronic Disease" makes it clear. They are not about curing disease, often not even about healthing disease, having given up on cures. They have adopted the assumption that chronic diseases are incurable and say so directly. *"Chronic diseases are long-lasting conditions that usually can be controlled but not cured."* As soon as you decide you cannot - you are right. The Center for Managing Chronic Disease cannot cure. Cure is not their name, not their game.

What does the Center for Managing Chronic Disease recommend? Manage the disease. Imagine if Cesar Millan came and saw your dog ripping your furniture to shreds, and he said *"buy cheap chairs made of steel, so the dog can't hurt it, you won't lose a lot of money. If you must be away during the daytime, give your dog sleeping pills, so he won't be running around the house wrecking things. If you can't control the dog, buy a sturdy collar and a short leash. Manage the disease."* It's the wrong solution for a chronic illness. Managing or medicating symptoms denies the existence of a cause, ignores the possibility of a cure.

Our medical systems are seldom interested in the present causes of a specific case of chronic illness. Causes are studied by epidemiologists, in statistical models, but not in real situations. Imagine you called Cesar Millan and told him your dog is barking all the time. Cesar lists of a statistical summary of the main reasons why your dog is barking all the time - maybe the dog hears lots of loud noises. Maybe the dog is nervous. Maybe another dog is barking. Maybe the dog is lonely. Statistics show each of these can contribute to a dog barking a lot. Maybe it's a combination of several causes. It's complicated. Then Cesar, if he were a medical doctor, might prescribe a medication. A tranquilizer to calm the dog. Ear plugs for the dog and the owner, and perhaps the neighbors as well. Doctor Cesar would not visit the home, observe the environment, the habits of the owner. He would not attempt to identify the present causes. The prescription should address causes, not the symptoms. Cesar cures, in part, by making house calls. Few doctors make house calls, and there are few cases where doctors diligently search for a cure cause.

When a chronic disease is judged, conventional medical practice seldom has intentions to cure. Assuming a cure is not possible, it aims for remission of symptoms. The results are predictable. No cures are found.

Our conventional medical systems claim to be scientific has a serious scientific flaw: ignorance of cures.

When a cure is attained, it's not noticed. Cesar has many successes - week after week we see new episodes, new cures. Cesar doesn't claim to cure. A doctor who claims a cure is dismissed as a quack. And a doctor who claimed as many cures as Cesar gives us in a month - would probably be banned from practice. In the past, he would be a saint - today he would be called a fraud, a huckster, his techniques labelled or branded a mixture of pseudoscience, snake oil and placebos. Medicine, our current system of modern medicine, does not count cures, does even not want cures, because few cures come from medicines. Cures come from health. Cures are ignored, dismissed, abolished or banned. Health is ignored.

And the result? Chronic diseases cannot be cured. The truth is a longer sentence.

Few chronic diseases can be cured by medicine.

When we study cures, we will learn that some attribute diseases can be cured by medicines, in some cases. Some chronic diseases are attribute diseases, which can be cured with medicines. But we cannot see these cases as cured until we take our studies of cure seriously.

Chronic diseases must be healthed one illness element at a time by addressing one chronic cause at a time, and healed as the healthing progresses. An illness is a hole in a healthiness. It can only be filled with health, not by medicines.

Circles of Illness, Causes, and Cures

A causal illness element has a present, active cause: a negative or unhealthy process. An injury illness element has a negative cause in the past. The injury is the present cause to be cured. An attribute illness element is caused by a negative attribute, a present cause. The attribute might have causes in the past, the present, and perhaps in the future.

> *This world and yonder world*
> *are incessantly giving birth:*
> *Every cause is a mother, its effect the child.*
> *When the effect is born, it too becomes a cause*
> *and gives birth to wondrous effects.*
> *These causes are generation on generation,*
> *but it needs a very well lighted eye*
> *to see the links in their chain.*
> *RUMI*

Rumi was not speaking about causes of illness, but the logic applies. Every cause has an effect: every effect becomes a cause, in healthiness, in illness, and in cures.

The Circle of Illness Elements

It's useful to view the three types of illness elements in a circle, which can also become a cycle or a downward spiral to unhealthiness, illness, disease, disability, and death.

This diagram illustrates the progressions of the three elements when they are not cured.

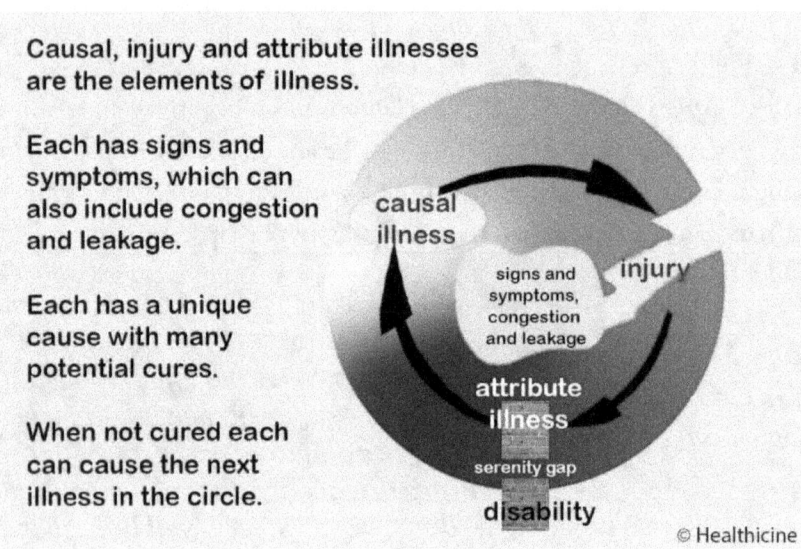

A causal illness might lead to an injury. An unhealed injury might become a negative attribute. A negative attribute can lead to causal illnesses, and new injuries. Causal illnesses, injuries, and attribute illnesses can lead to congestion or leakage in body, mind, spirit, or community. A cure might cause additional cures or illnesses. A transformation cure often creates an injury illness, requiring a healing cure, which might lead to or facilitate a causal cure. Sometimes cures lead to illness, and sometimes illnesses lead to cures.

Injuries and attribute illnesses that are not cured can lead to disability. The *serenity gap* is the distance between an attribute illness caused by a negative attribute which can be transformed and a disability, as in the serenity prayer:

> *God grant me the serenity to accept the things I cannot change; courage to change the things I can; and wisdom to know the difference.*
> *- Reinhold Niebuhr*

An attribute illness can be cured. A disability cannot be cured. Sometimes an injury cannot be healed, or the cause of a causal illness cannot be addressed. The gap between a curable illness and disability depends on our spirits, our ability to cure, and our belief that we can or cannot cure.

The Circle of Causes

We can expand the circle of elements of illness to create a circle of causes. Congestion can be a cause of illness, not just a symptom. The circle of causes contains the circle of illnesses because many illnesses are causes of illness.

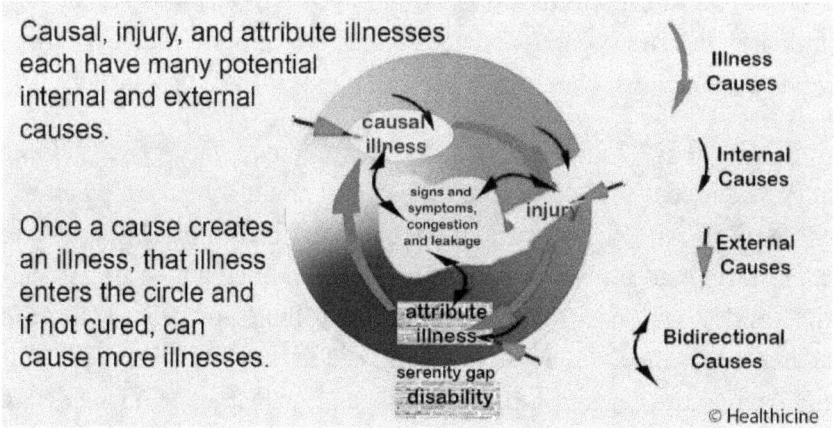

The circle of potential causes is full of arrows.

> *Life don't clickety-clack down a straight-line track*
> *It comes together and it comes apart.*
> --- Ferron

Many internal processes and forces can cause illness. Many external processes and forces can cause illness. Healthiness has many internal and external boundaries. Every cause is part of a chain of causes. To cure, we must focus attention on a specific cause, a cause that cures. Each cause, and each link in a present causal chain provides opportunities to cure.

Internally caused illnesses are prevented and cured by improving internal healthiness. Externally caused illnesses might be prevented and cured by improving internal or external healthiness. The best cures come from health, not from medicines.

The Circle of Cures

The circle of cures reverses the arrows of the circle of illness. A complex illness with a single primary cause might consist of a causal illness, resulting in injuries, which lead to an attribute illness, requiring three types of cure actions.

Curing proceeds by addressing a present cause. The causal illness element is cured, or stopped when the causal chain is broken, when the cause is addressed. Healing cures injury illnesses. Healing is always active, before, during, and after an illness, and can be encouraged or assisted with healthy actions. Transforming cures illnesses caused by the presence or absence of a negative attribute. The attribute illness element is cured when the negative attribute has been transformed, and necessary healing has completed. If the illness has created or become a disability, that cannot be cured.

The Elements of Curing

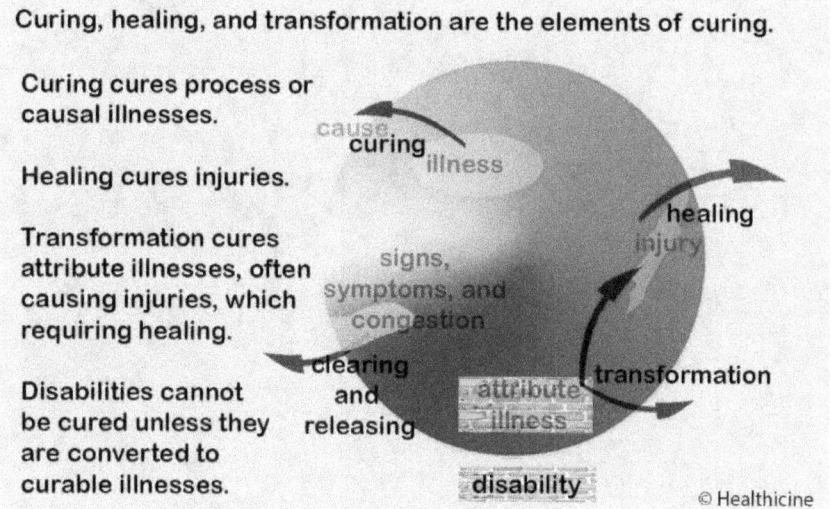

Curing, healing, and transformation are the elements of curing.

Curing cures process or causal illnesses.

Healing cures injuries.

Transformation cures attribute illnesses, often causing injuries, which requiring healing.

Disabilities cannot be cured unless they are converted to curable illnesses.

If congestion or leakage is present, it should also be cleared. As cures progress, the illness elements fade, signs and symptoms of the illness element fade and disappear. It is possible, sometimes necessary to work on elementary cures in specific sequences. However, when a prior illness in the circle is not cured, the subsequent illness element might continue or reoccur.

Many illnesses cause injuries or negative attributes. Sometimes a causal illness causes an injury, or a negative attribute, and is then cured by natural healthiness – but an injury or a negative attribute remains. If only an injury remains – only healing is required. When a negative attribute remains, causing further illness, a transformation is required.

A disease cure often consists of several sets of cures for a set of complex and compound illnesses elements. Each elementary cure is unique to an illness element. Every disease or complex illness cure is unique to the case. Every cure is an anecdote, a personal story, a personal success. Many disease cures are stories with many parts, a series of anecdotes, which we can only begin to understand as we study cures.

Every illness has a cause. Every cure has a cause – we call these causes *"cures."*

Cured

We can summarize of illnesses and cures:

An illness element is cured when its present cause and consequences have been successfully addressed.

- **an illness element** is an illness or component of an illness, having a single or elementary present cause or causal chain. An illness element can have many negative consequences, including signs and symptoms, injuries, negative attribute consequences, and even other illnesses. The cause of an illness might come from diet, body, mind, spirit, community, or the environment. A causal chain can link from one area to another. The negative consequences of an illness can affect body, mind, spirit, community and environment.

There are three types of illness elements,
- A **causal illness element** has a present process or absence of process cause and is cured by addressing the causal chain.
- An **injury illness element** consists of damage, the cause is gone. Injuries, injury illness elements, are cured by healing.
- An **attribute illness element** is caused by the presence or absence of an attribute and cured by transformation, by transforming the cause to a neutral or positive attribute.

A **compound illness** is an illness with multiple present causes, possibly multiple causal chains, consisting of a set of elementary or complex illnesses with different causes, and similar or overlapping consequences. Many diseases, even many cases of diseases that are simple in theory, are compound illnesses. Compound illnesses are cured one illness element at a time.

A **complex illness** consists of a set of multiple illness elements with a single causal chain. Complex illnesses are cured one illness element at a time.

A **chronic illness** is has a chronic present cause. A chronic illness element might be a causal illness, an injury illness, or an attribute illness. Causal chronic illnesses have a chronic process cause. Chronic injury illnesses are complex because the cause is still present and active – sometimes another illness. Attribute illnesses are naturally chronic because they are caused by things that exist over time. Chronic illnesses are cured by addressing the chronic attribute of the cause. They often require addressing the consequences of the cause and the cure. When chronic illnesses are not cured, they often grow in severity and accumulate causes.

Incurable: that which cannot be cured is not a curable illness. It might be a negative attribute that cannot be transformed, a disability or handicap, or perhaps a natural feature, to be accepted, but not cured.

> *Complete freedom from disease and from struggle is almost incompatible with the process of living.*
> *--- Rene Dubos*

What Happens After a Cure?

Today, when a cure occurs, it is ignored. The patient might celebrate, the doctor might nod, but that's it. The illness is cured. Patients and doctors who claim cured are generally ignored, there being no definition of cured, there can be no proof.

Sometimes, cures are represented in case studies, when a specific case is unique and illustrates some complex analysis, but the word cure is generally avoided in favor of treatments.

What Should Happen after a Cure?

If we are to be serious and scientific about cures, we need to study them scientifically. We need to recognize, scientifically, that every illness has many potential cures, and that the cure proves the cause.

A case diagnosed as arthritis might be cured by diet in one case, by exercise in another, and by a medicine the promotes healing in another. A case diagnosed as heart disease might be cured by diet, exercise, or both. The cure identifies the cause.

A chronic disease might be cured by a transformation of mind, or spirit, or by a surgery or lesser disruption followed by healing. The cure proves the cause.

When we study cures, we might begin to see them everywhere, to demystify them, even to understand miracle cures.

Hypothetical Case Study: Food Poisoning

Using our new understanding of the elements of cure, and the concepts of cures, curing, and cured, let's look at an illness that is simple in theory, to explore these concepts further:

Terry has been working hard all day and has come home to dinner, proudly prepared by little Terry. Terry eats a large bowl of chili and gets a case of food poisoning. There are symptoms at both ends, throwing up, and diarrhea, resulting in soreness in the mouth and itching at the other end. After several hours, Terry recovers from the food poisoning, without visiting a doctor. The itchiness heals over a few days. But there's a residual problem, a negative mental or spirit blockage. Terry no longer eats chili. The very smell of chili makes Terry sick. This might not be a problem. But, Terry's family and Terry's communities love chili. They make and eat chili a lot. Over the course of several months, Terry becomes more and more accustomed to the smell and look of chili. Gradually, Terry tastes a bit of chili and learns to enjoy it again. Terry's cure is now complete.

This story illustrates many important aspects of cause and cure.

What was the cause of Terry's illness?

First, we need to recognize that Terry had and cured, three elements of illness, with three cures. There was the food poisoning was an attribute illness, caused by the unhealthy chili, cured by healthy vomiting and diarrhea. There was the injury illness, caused by the food poisoning illness, was cured by healing. There was the blockage attribute illness in the mind, by understanding the source and the memories of illness, and the spirits – the desire to not get sick again. The blockage attribute illness element was cured by a transformation that took place gradually, assisted by a healthy community.

What caused the unhealthy chili? Was it caused by little-Terry's inattention or lack of understanding of how to make healthy chili? Was it caused by poor instructions or training? Or was it caused by unhealthy meat or other ingredients in the chili? If so, what was the cause of the unhealthiness of the ingredients? These are explanatory causes, preventative causes, perhaps *blame causes* in a past causal chain, but they cannot cure. They are not cure causes. The illness has been cured.

We often search for the cause of a cause, and the cause of a cause – never reaching a root cause – in our desire to prevent future illnesses. Only cure causes lead to cures when illness is present.

The tainted quality of the food was an attribute that caused a poisoning illness and the injury illnesses. These led to the blockage illness, an illness of mind and spirit. Sometimes a bad reaction to a food can lead to positive preventative actions, sometimes to negative avoidance.

Every case of an illness is unique. A minor food poisoning might only progress to a single causal illness. A more serious case results in injury illnesses. When the case is very severe – an attribute illness can also result. Only rare and severe cases cause to death.

Studying the chain of illness elements helps us to understand the illnesses which were cured by health, not by medicines.

The cause of Terry's illness was addressed by healthiness, by the ejection of the toxic chili, without medical intervention. This was a temporary (from the perspective of a life form that can eject the poison) attribute cause.

Healing injuries caused by the illness began as soon as the body noticed the injuries and continued for a few days until healing of the injury elements was completed.

The blockage illness transformation occurred gradually over several weeks after the food poisoning illness was cured and healing completed. In this case, the negative attribute was removed by Terry's communities and there was no need for healing after the transformation.

Most cases of food poisoning, even those causing permanent damage or death, are viewed as single diseases by conventional medicine. There is no test for cured for food poisoning. Most medical case studies are short term and fail to see the chili eating blockage as an illness, much less notice its cure. When several illnesses are present, several cures are necessary. Conventional medicine sees a single disease and then fails to comprehend all three cures as cures.

More complex diseases, consisting of compound illnesses with multiple causes might require a complex analysis for each cause. It's not worthwhile to study every case with this amount of rigor – but it is necessary to study enough cases to gain a general understanding.

The analysis of illness elements and chains of causes make more illness visible – enabling more cures. When only the disease view is used, individual cures can't be seen even when they occur and the disease cure is lost in the confusion.

A severe case of depression, for example, might have multiple causes. A simple depression illnesses might be cured as naturally as a sliver or a paper cut, although perhaps requiring more time. In the 1960s, depression was widely considered curable – but today, cured is not defined for depression. Depression that is easily cured is often excluded from the definition of depression as a disease. Conventional medicine has moved beyond studies of simple cures to only recognizing and approving complex disease treatments that do not cure.

Case Study: Transformation

About 20 years ago, I began to experience numbness in the fingers of my left hand. It started slowly in my little finger, and slowly progressed across my hand. I went to a conventional medical clinic, where the doctor made a minor examination and suggested a wrist brace and *"perhaps a massage treatment would help"* – he did not recommend a therapist.

I did some research and found a massage therapist who had also studied osteopathy, acupuncture, and other treatment and healing modalities. Let's call her Lydia (not her real name).

Lydia began by examining my hand and arm, carefully and thoroughly. She advised me that the treatment might take several visits and did not use the word cure. She massaged my hand and wrist aggressively and said there would be some symptoms of healing. When I left, my hand felt a bit better, but only a bit. I booked a treatment next week.

The next week, Lydia examined my hand again and started working on my forearm. I was a bit confused. She said – *"the hand is not the problem. It's farther up. We need to work backwards to find the source."* She massaged the hand again, and then she pushed hard at a point on my forearm, just before the elbow. It hurt, and she warned me, *"If it doesn't hurt, it won't be much use. It will feel better after it heals."*

Over the course of several weeks, Lydia worked her way up my arm, into my shoulder. She explained that she was releasing *"knots"* (blockages) and then giving me a week to heal, and then progressing further. My hand was getting better – I felt cured, but she warned me that the source had not yet been found.

Then one day, after several weeks, she quickly checked by hand, my forearm, upper arm, shoulder, and started working down my back. *"That's it"* she exclaimed proudly. *"We've found it."* She began to massage an area in my lower back.

As she prodded, I had a flashback.

About eight months before, on a beautiful summer day, I had taken an all-day bike ride. I like to ride – but normally I ride an hour or so. On this day, I rode for seven or eight hours and arrived home feeling great, and exhausted.

The next morning, I could not stand up. I crawled out of bed to get to the bathroom. I gradually recovered enough to get into the car and drive to a medical clinic. The doctor prescribed muscle relaxants and sent me home. The muscle relaxants helped with the pain – I don't like painkillers, so I took only a few. After a few days I felt better.

Muscle relaxants helped me feel better but did nothing to address the damage done to the tissues in my back. The damage was healed, but the healing was faulty, leaving an invisible physical blockage, a negative attribute.

Over the course of eight months, the damage caused a chain of minor blockage illnesses, which I did not notice, until it surfaced in my hand, as tension and numbness.

Lydia did not search for the root cause – the biking, my bike, my posture, the muscle relaxants, or failure to cure. She searched for the root illness, not the root cause.

She worked slowly, transforming the chain of illnesses in my hand, my forearm, my upper arm, shoulder, back, and lower back. Each transformation required some healing, and testing, sometimes repeating next week to ensure that it was complete. When she reached my lower back, Lydia knew she had found the root illness. She asked me to book another appointment for an examination but did not expect any more problems.

Today, 20 years later, the problem has not reappeared. A forceful transformation cured it, although much gentler than any surgery, and much more effectively.

To Have an Illness, or To Be Ill

We easily slip between two concepts of illness, without much thought. Sometimes we see ourselves as *having an illness*. I have a cold. When I was young, I had measles. Other times, we use words that suggest we are ill, or that we are the illness. We might say *"I am a diabetic."* But we might also say *"I have diabetes."* We might suggest, or argue, that one view is more accurate than another. After all, no illness is a *thing* – except for injuries. We cannot *have* an illness, nor can we g*et rid of* an illness. On the other hand, saying that we are an illness, as in *"I am a diabetic"* is not accurate either. We might say *"I am ill"* in the sense that we might say *"I am sad"* or *"I am happy,"* to describe how we feel.

How we view cured, depends on our view of healthiness and our view of illness. When we see ourselves as *"having an illness,"* we want to get rid of the illness. The having view promotes medical approaches. We want to buy a medicine to cure the illness. When we are cured, we believe the medicine cured the illness.

When we see ourselves as *"being ill"* we can recognize that illness, like healthiness, is part of ourselves, part of our health. We are our health; we are our illness. The being view promotes healthy approaches, recognizes that to be cured, we must change. The *"being ill"* view advises us that buying or taking medicines is unlikely to cure.

These distinctions are important. Different views, different concepts of illness lead us to different cure actions. Consciously choosing between these two views can help us find more cures, to cure more effectively.

When we wish to cure an illness, we can only succeed by addressing the cause and healing the damage. Do we cure by having a cure, or by being cured? No medicine can cure any illness without an action. We might cure bacterial infection by taking a medicine that kills the bacteria.

Antibiotics only cure when they are taken, in specific doses, for a specific illness. Every cure is an action, not a physical thing, not a pill.

Killing the cause only works for an illness we see as caused by a pathogen. We can buy cures for a few infectious illnesses. However, this is not always the most effective cure, even for many illnesses we view as caused by pathogens. A chronic infection can only be cured by health. No medicine can cure *chronic*.

When we view an illness as caused by a thing – bacteria – we cure by killing the bacteria, an attribute caused the illness. If we cure a similar illness by improving the health of the patient, which fights off the infection, we view the illness as a causal illness, caused by a lack of healthiness. Which view is right? The right view is proven by the cure.

The cure defines the cause.

We cannot buy cures for most diseases. We sometimes treat deficiency illnesses, by buying something to address the current state of deficiency, but a cure requires addressing the deficiency on an ongoing basis, not just treating its present state. We cannot buy a cure for any illness caused by an excess, like heart diseases, obesity or diabetes. Most of the time, when we buy a medicine, it does not cure, because our illnesses are part of us, part of our lives, not something we can buy or kill. Most medicines treat signs and symptoms of illness while ignoring cause.

An illness is a hole in a healthiness. When we are ill, we have a hole in our healthiness, which cannot be filled with medicines, it can only be filled with health. Medicines might hide the hole, or help us to forget the hole, but they can't fill the hole. A curable illness is a judgement that an illness exists and that it can be cured. Most illnesses are cured with health, by improving healthiness.

Health is the best cure, the only true cure. We cannot buy health, but we might have it. We might be a picture of health, when we study cures.

Summary and Conclusions

> *Health is whole.*
> *Health is wide and deep.*
> *Health is slow and steady.*
> *Health is honest and true.*
> *Health is the best preventative.*
> *Health is the best cure, the only true cure.*
> *The Healthicine Creed*

Cures come from Health

All cures come from health. There are no *health tricks*. We cannot trick health. Illness is caused by a lack of healthiness, cured by improving healthiness.

A causal cure addresses present illness element, with a present cause. Causal cures are healthy cures, accomplished by improving the health of the patient. A cure might be aided by healthy actions of the patient or the community. Causal illnesses can usually be traced to some action or inaction of the patient, like a faulty diet, exercise, or rest pattern. Most causal illnesses are cured naturally, by the health of the patient, sometimes before we become conscious of them. No medicine can change the life activities of a patient.

Only healing can cure an injury illness. Healing is part of growth, always active, even when no illness is present, facilitated and aided by healthiness, by proper diet, by physical, mental, spirit, and community exercise and rest, healthiness, and support. The immune system is a healing system and a powerful curing system.

Transformation is change, sometimes coming about when the patient becomes aware of a negative attribute and changes themselves. We often fear change, and rightfully so. Change can cure, but change can also cause illness. Changes that cure might also create significant distress as the cure progresses. On the other hand, sometimes a transformational cure comes about without awareness. We might notice that a problem "went away" without any conscious action. A friend might observe and say, *"you've changed,"* to your surprise. Transformations can also be induced with the help of an external person, or by physical, mental, spirit, or community actions that consciously or unconsciously change a negative attribute, curing an illness.

Medicating Signs and Symptoms

Conventional medicine sells treatments, preferably those that can be packaged and delivered via the patent protection of a doctor's prescription, and function without human intervention. Treatments are often *things* that can receive FDA approval. But healthiness and illnesses are processes, not things. Few treatments can cure. Even an antibiotic must be part of a process. It must be consumed on schedule. Too much can be toxic, too little, ineffective. Most conventional and most alternative medicines make no attempt to cure. The enormous success of antibiotics has resulted in many cures. But this success has made us lazy, searching for medicines to cure diseases which cannot be cured with medicines. Perhaps success has also led to our failure to understand cures. Most people and many doctors mistakenly believe a medicine is necessary to cure.

We often prefer to have – to buy a cure, over being cured. Cures might put responsibility on the patient, where it often belongs. But doctors and pharmaceutical companies cannot package and sell *being cured.* Attempts to purchase a cure lead to purchases of non-cures, and ongoing searches for new non-cure treatments.

It is easy to treat one illness while increasing the risk of another, when we place all attention on treatments and ignore cures.

Conventional medicines, except for anti-parasitic medicines, rarely cure. Most are symptomicines, advertised to address signs and symptoms, with no intention to cure. Cures come from health.

Preventatives

We often hear statements like *"prevention is the best medicine,"* or *"prevention is better than cure."* These phrases are simplistic. Will our insurance pay for the best medicine? Insurance companies pay for treatments on their list, like vaccines, but will not pay for healthy preventatives. They will not pay for cures either – unless they are on the list. And cures, named as such, are not on their lists.

Any illness caused by another illness is best prevented with a cure. Health is the best preventative and the best cure. Chronic diseases are often best prevented by curing the illness before it is a diagnosable disease, or before it becomes chronic.

Preventatives are not always healthy, but health is always a preventative. Many preventative cures are speculative, containing significant risk. Preventatives seldom cure illnesses in the present. Some speak of preventatives as curing future illnesses, but these illnesses are speculative, not yet real. Conventional medicine marketers love preventatives – they can sell without any hint of curing. In some cases, they are important, in other cases, they are supported by marketing mantras or promotion of beliefs that are not studied scientifically. Is fluoride the best preventative for tooth decay? There are no studies searching for the best preventative of dental disease. There is no interest. Fluoride has strengths and weaknesses, but fluoride is a marketable product approved by the FDA. There is no market incentive to find anything better, even to decide which situations warrant fluoride, and which do not. Doing so will decrease sales. Selling fluoride is big business. Searching for, even acknowledging the possibility of better alternatives puts business at risk.

It is possible to prevent illness by never taking any risks, by decreasing healthiness. Crossing the street might lead to injury, disability, and even death. But choosing never to cross the street is not the best medicine. It diminishes healthiness. Walk, don't run. Crossing at the crosswalk, after looking out for traffic, is a healthy preventative.

Cures come from health, not from preventatives.

Visualizing Cures

We can represent the concepts of illness, from causes to cures in a single diagram:

A Calculus of Curing

cause — healthiness — cure

process, force, attribute → causal illness, injury illness, attribute illness → cure, heal, transform

illness © Healthicine

Every illness has a cause. Every cause is a process cause (an active process or absence of process over time, a verb), a force cause (a stress or absence of stress) or an attribute cause (a something or absence of something that results in illness, a noun). These three types of causes produce three distinct types of illnesses, respectively: causal illnesses, injury illnesses, and attribute illnesses. The three types of illness are cured by different types of cure actions, respectively: causal cures (cures), healing cures (healing) and transformational cures (transformations).

Every illness is a result of a decrease in healthiness and often a cause of further decreases in healthiness. Each elementary cause of illness results in a single instance of illness. When the cause is repeating, causes a repeating illness. When the cause is chronic, it causes a chronic illness.

Health is the best cure. Healthiness is also the best preventative. The cure for any illness is an improvement in health, a specific kind of healthiness for each type of illness. When we raise a specific kind of healthiness, we reduce a corresponding unhealthiness, and illnesses are cured.

Every true cure is an improvement in healthiness. How many diseases are best cured by health? When we make cures our goal, all of them. If they can be cured, they can only be cured by health. Even an incurable condition is best treated with healthiness. We might find it cured.

We need to spend more time, energy and money pursuing cures, and less pursuing treatments, patents, and profits, with no intention to cure.

There is much to study, much to learn about cures. Many important cures have been discovered again and again, but are ignored, even denied - because they are not marketable products. Conventional medicine has many discoveries or *"half invented"* products, to use a phrase from Nassim Nicholas Taleb. Discovered, and rediscovered many times. They are difficult, or impossible, to bring to market. How far is the distance from medical theory to medical practice? Six inches – the length of the almighty dollar. If it doesn't make money, if it doesn't provide patent protection, it's impossible to control sales, so no one will sell it, and as a result, no one can buy it. Many cures cannot be bought at all. You can't buy *eating less*. Your insurance won't pay for it even if it cures.

At present, *"health care"* is a marketing euphemism for illness care. No health clinic cares for us when we are healthy. Illness, curable illnesses, might be present long before a specific disease can be diagnosed. No insurance will pay for treatments, nor cures without a diagnosis of disease.

Today, many cases of disease are diagnosed without analysis of present cause. Even the latest medical fashions like Science Based Medicine, and Functional Medicine are technically ignorant of present cause and of the chronic attribute of causes of chronic diseases. Neither contains a useful definition of cure, much less chronic cure. There are few cures recognized – phrases like recovery, reversal, remission are preferred. Even when a cure is encountered, it is seldom recognized as a cure. Treatments for signs and symptoms are designed, tested, manufactured, approved by governments, recommended, and sold without intention to cure. Symptomicines, although they make no attempt to cure, can be useful to provide relief of symptoms. They sometimes reduce risk but do not cure. Symptomicines often helps us forget illness, encouraging us to ignore cures, as illness continues and grows, as causes accumulate.

Only a specific illness can be cured, in a specific patient, one illness element at a time. Every patient is unique. Each patient has unique causal chains of illness. Every illness is unique. Every cure is unique in some ways, sometimes even for the same disease in the same patient at a later time in their life.

When we study of elements of illness, elements of cause, chains of cause, and develop a calculus of curing, we can learn to take simple diseases apart, and cure them regularly, in most cases without medicines. We can begin to learn about curable illnesses, incurable conditions, and to understand the fundamental difference between illness and chronic illness.

We can begin with simple illness elements, learn to cure and to understand simple cures. Over time, we can build our understanding and technique to encompass more complex illnesses and diseases, more complex cures.

We will not begin to succeed until we begin to cure.

> *We have not succeeded in answering all our problems — indeed we sometimes feel we have not completely answered any of them. The answers we have found have only served to raise a whole set of new questions. In some ways we feel that we are as confused as ever, but we think we are confused on a higher level and about more important things. The Workshop Way of Learning*
> *- Earl C. Kelley*

To find cures, we must define cured for every illness element. We must build a definition of cured for each case of a disease. To learn to cure, we must practice curing and practice judging cured. Most current treatments are distractions, ignorant of cures.

We need to move beyond *"the cure,"* beyond the naive belief that every illness, every disease has only one cure. We need to move forward through many cures, to search for better cures. Every illness has many opportunities to cure; each cure has strengths and weaknesses. Some cures are better for some patients in some cases. Other cures might be better for other patients, or at other times. Some cures are faster, some more reliable, some more effective. To find the best for each case, we need to move away from the bureaucracies of conventional medicine.

Until we accept the possibility of many cures for every illness, we cannot begin to explore the many dimensions of curing.

In the final analysis, we will learn that we cannot change our illnesses without changing ourselves, because every illness is a part of our lives, part of our healthiness, part of ourselves.

We cure by changing ourselves, by changing our lives, our health, our bodies, minds, spirits, communities and environments. We cure by becoming healthier. We cannot become healthier with treatments that make us feel better with our diseases, nor treatments that help us to *"live with our disease,"* only with cures.

It's time for a science of medicine. And a science of cures.

To your health, tracy
Founder: Healthicine

Every illness can be cured. The Healthicine Creed

Epilogue: Books That Cure

There are thousands of books claiming to cure. Can you name one that is generally accepted and supported by our current medical establishment? I can't. Most, perhaps all are simply ignored. How can this be? Why does it happen? Does conventional medicine suffer a total ignorance of cures?

As we have learned, cure, curing, cures, and cured are poorly defined in conventional medicine, if they are defined at all. The words cure and treatment –are often used without any distinction between the two.

Cure: When many people think of a cure, they see a cure as the end of an illness, a disease, a medical condition, even a disability where medicine is no longer required. We see lots of chronic diseases, which cannot be cured by medicines, so it's easy to assume there are lots of incurable diseases. Our powerful medical systems are awash with incurable diseases, without definitions of cure or incurable.

Treatment: Many dictionaries define cure as *"a treatment"* with little respect to effectiveness. Many books with cure in the title, are about treatments which make no attempt to cure. The advice often presented is to *"learn to live with your disease,"* as if there are no cures. The recommendation might be reworded as *"learn to die with your disease."* in the interest of honesty.

Books about curing illness seldom use the word cure in the title or the contents. The word cure is forbidden in medicine. Cures are miracles – and we cannot study miracles with science. Anyone who claims to cure is accused of lying or suspected of being a witch or demon, a quack, or a huckster.

Can we find books that cure? My local library lists 297 books about diabetes, a search on Amazon for *"cure diabetes"* produces over 600.

They range from Fun To Know facts about Diabetes, to Yoga for Diabetes, to The American Diabetes Association Complete Guide to Diabetes offers *"offers expert advice to diabetics on living an active, healthy life,"* but no cure. Are there any with advice on how to cure diabetes? Yes. I've found a few. I'm certain there are more. Of course, if you find one, it doesn't necessarily mean you can cure your diabetes—any more than finding a book about building a house means you can build your house. But if you don't find one, your chances of a cure are much lower. Conventional medicine views diabetes as an incurable disease. Most books about diabetes, including many with cure in the title, contain no definition of cure, offer no cures, and no hope for cures.

To cure illness, we need more than books. We need to understand what is meant by cure. We might also need assistance. Many books that cure are supported by single doctors or small organizations offering help you cure your illness. But can they cure?

Can you name an organization, recognized by the conventional medical establishment, that helps people to cure a disease? I can't. No one claims to cure. Cure is a four-letter word. Forbidden.

Can Books Cure?

No book can cure any disease. To cure is to address the cause. No book, by itself, can address the cause of an illness. A book can only point the way. The cure is up to the patient. Curing, in most cases, is a DIY (Do It Yourself) Project.

To cure any illness with a book, we must take some specific actions recommended by the book. Illness elements are cured by health, by healthy actions. However, many health actions can be dangerous. Actions that move healthiness in one direction can also move another healthiness in a different direction.

Do any books really cure? Do any books lead to cures? Can you name a single book that documents how to cure? Who can you ask? No one. There is no medical definition of cured, no scientific or medical organization to define cure, no organization that tests and validates cures – with the possible exception of the doctors at Lourdes. No one tests cure claims to determine when they are valid. Cures don't count. Conventional medicine counts diseases and causes of death. No one counts cures. There are no statistics for cures.

There are lots of people and lots of organizations claiming X is not a cure, few who will claim Y is a cure. No one can give a scientific analysis of any cure claim, except for illnesses caused by pathogens. We can search for a medical authority on cures and cured. There are none. There are no medical journals interested in publishing cures. Medical journals publish clinical studies of treatments, in most cases, treatments that make no attempt to define cure, much less to cure.

This list is a first step, a small list of books that cure. I hope it will open a discussion, and spur scientific analysis. I'm not holding my breath.

I list books that cure. These are only a few of the books of which I am aware. Someday, when we begin to study cures with science, many books will be recognized as valuable guides to curing illness.

I have listed books by the type of cure, by the type of illness element cured – causal, injury, and attribute, and the three corresponding types of cures – causal, healing, transformation. The concept of an element of illness does not exist in conventional medicine today, and as a result, it does not appear in any of the books that cure. However, when we look closely, we often see books that cure recommending actions for specific illness elements, not for diseases.

Every cure, every action that cures, does so by improving the health of the patient. Most, perhaps all books that cure, do so by improving healthiness.

Curing (Causal Cures)

Curing an active causal illness is accomplished by addressing the cause, the present causal chains, of the illness. A chronic illness has an additional layer of cause, the chronic attribute of a cause. Many active illnesses are cured by addressing the activity, or absence of activity leading to the illness. The patient becomes healthier as the illness fades away.

Many of these books recommend a shotgun technique. Many different actions are used at once, to improve the health of the patient. It may be possible, but not necessarily easier, to cure the illness with fewer changes. The shotgun technique has a high rate of success because it implements many health improvements at once. A cure is a cure. Nobody complains if the patient's health was improved in unnecessary ways. The side effects of health cures are healthy.

Improving healthiness can be challenging work. A cure for a chronic illness requires change to life's processes, or a physical, mental, spirit, or community change. Change is hard. It might take many changes to attain a complete cure of a complex illness. A coach, a mentor, or a buddy might be critical to cure success. Few doctors are ready to coach patients to a cure. Coaching takes time, and time – especially medical time – is expensive. Medical doctors are trained to treat illness, not to cure.

However, cures are possible, commonplace even. Here are some of my favorite books that cure.

Cure Tooth Decay: Heal and Prevent Cavities with Nutrition by Ramiel Nagel and Timothy Gallagher

This is the first book I remember seeing that has cure in the title – and dares to advise how to cure in the contents. It is often dismissed or shunned for that reason alone. A book about curing illnesses of the teeth, gums, and mouth, it pulls no punches. These illnesses are cured by health, healthy foods, healthy eating, and healthy eating exercises.

Cure Tooth Decay cures causal illnesses and injury illnesses. It addresses illness by cause in ways that promote healing. I highly recommend this book to anyone as a starter for learning about cures and about dental health.

It is also a powerful book about prevention of illness. The best cure is health. Health is the best preventative. It is interesting to compare the recommendations in this book, with regards to prevention – to those of a conventional dentist. It quickly becomes clear that many current dental recommendations offer little to improve healthiness. They are designed to be sold for a profit.

The book does not mention dental surgery cures. It does not recognize transformation as a cure. Dentists often cure attribute illnesses by surgical transformation. Like many books, it often uses the word healing even when transformation is more accurate. Healing transforms – so it's easy to assume, in error, that all transformations are a result of healing.

Radical Remission: Surviving Cancer Against All Odds by Kelly A. Turner PhD

Kelly A Turner's research led her to study thousands of people who *"put their cancer into remission."* Cured is not defined for cancer and cannot be proven. Turner avoids the word cure. Her research identified nine key factors for curing cancer. Each improves healthiness, in separate ways, addressing many possible causes of illness at once. It's a shotgun technique that can be used to cure many different illnesses, not just cancers.

Although she seldom uses the forbidden word cure, Turner closes with

"Curing means getting rid of a disease, while healing means becoming whole. Curing is sometimes possible, while healing is always possible."

Can you use Dr. Turner's approach to cure your cancer? Health is slow and many cancers proceed slowly. However, Unfortunately, many cancers are diagnosed very late – at the point where danger is severe. Even minor cancers are often treated as if they were emergencies, prompting the patient to undertake faster treatments. I am not a doctor, and I don't have cancer, but if I did, I would go back and read this book again before any other actions.

A Mind of Your Own: The Truth About Depression and How Women Can Heal Their Bodies to Reclaim Their Lives by Kelly Brogan, M.D., Kristin Loberg

Depression is classified as incurable (by lack of definition of cured) in current conventional medical practice. This is a relatively new situation – 50 years ago most cases of depression were considered curable. Today's conventional medicine has progressed such that depression is defined as a treatable *symptom domain*. Conventional medicine does not use the word cure for any mental illness – depression is no exception.

Depression can have a physical cause, from nutritional deficiencies to toxic excesses, including drugs. It can also be an illness of the mind, a metaphysical illness, which cannot be cured with physical methods. We can induce depression by depressing the spirits, by putting a prisoner into solitary confinement, depriving them of community interactions, driving them to depression. A single patient might suffer many different depression illnesses at once, which medical practice diagnoses as a single disease. Depression is generally treated without reference to cause. When cause is ignored, several illness elements accumulate and are diagnosed as a single disease. Cures become impossible.

Kelly, like most authors, avoids the word cure, but many of her case studies are clearly cures – even though cured is not defined. Kelly's patients are often cured using a shotgun technique, consisting of many changes completed over time to improve many healthinesses – physical, mental, spirit, and community. Depression fades away as healthiness rises.

There is no medical technique to diagnose depression cured. Our conventional medical establishment ignores claims of depression cured. We count deaths, suicides, caused by depression, but not cures. We count failures while ignoring successes.

The Depression Cure by Dr. Stephen S. Ilhardi

According to the Depression Cure, depression has six basic causes. Dr. Ilardi doesn't give them specific names, so I've created cause names. I've put Ilardi's wording in brackets followed by a clarification:

- Diet (dietary omega three fatty acids -deficiency or imbalance)
- Mind and Spirit (engaging activity – lack of balance – rumination)
- Exercise of Body (physical exercise – lack of)
- Sunlight (sunlight – lack of)
- Community (social support – lack of or negative)
- Sleep and Rest (sleep – lack of)

Dr. Ilardi uses the word cure in the book title but tends to avoid the word cure in the text, apologizing with *"The Depression Cure. Admittedly this is a bold title."* and closing the book with the hopeful *"We can live the depression cure."*

Dr. Ilardi's book gives detailed descriptions of each cause and provides prescriptions for curing. None of the cures are medicines.

The Bloat Cure: 101 Natural Solutions for Real and Lasting Relief by Robynne Chutkan

The bloat cure presents one short article at a time, 101 different present causes (although that term is not used), therefore 101 different types of bloat illness and 101 different cure actions. We can view each cause and associated consequences as an illness element – although the authors do not use that term.

Bloat is not generally considered a disease. The ICD10 lists *"abdominal distension (gaseous),"* but bloating is generally considered a symptom of another condition, not a disease. Major medical references make no mention of cure with regards to bloating or abdominal distension. It's not a disease, and there is no cure. It appears to be not important that any female of a certain age is familiar with bloat, if not in her own body, in discussions with friends. Officially, it's not in the book. It's not in the ICD10 list of disease codes – it's a symptom without a disease.

The book uses the word cure rarely, although I am certain it can help people to cure many bloat illness elements. There is a cure technique referenced twice in the book, a shotgun technique to improve the health of the patient, which will cure a bloat illness element caused by one or more of the items addressed by the shotgun technique.

Unfortunately, the book is presented in alphabetical sequence by cause, making it difficult to read and to use as a DIY cure source. It's a list book, designed to attract attention to "101 cures" rather than a recipe book that might be used to cure individual cases of illness effectively. I believe the authors could, with a little effort, produce a more effective DIY book to cure bloat, that recommends an effective sequence of questions and actions.

The New Rational Manager by Charles Higgins Kepner, Benjamin B. Tregoe

This is not a medical book, but it illustrates many keys to cure. The Kepner-Tregoe system for problem-solving and decision making provides powerful techniques to identify the cause of a problem and to choose alternative ways to address the problem and to prevent future problems. It clearly acknowledges that addressing problems requires analysis of cause, generation and analysis of alternative actions and that success indicates that the problem has been resolved (cured). It is written for managers, but the techniques are generic, and can also be used to find, test, and manage cures for illnesses. The book does not use the word cure at all. It is not a medical text. Rather, it is a book about managing problematical causes and effects. It is a very powerful general cure technique for many business problems.

In their quest to produce a general system to resolve complex problems, simple problems being easily resolved, the authors missed some essential basics of problem solving. The book has no concept of an elementary problem, and elementary cause, and no concept of a present cause.

Healing (Injury Cures)

Many books with cure in the title are about healing cures. Our bodies, minds, spirits, and communities are experienced in healing themselves. Healing is an important cure. There are lots of books in this field, and it can be difficult to separate the wheat from the chaff. There are many books about mysteries and mysticism of healing. Healing is magic in many ways, but not mystical. I believe that much of the mysticism around curing comes from confusing transformations and healing. Transformations are mystical.

Doctor's don't heal – only patients can heal – but a doctor's actions and recommendations can promote efficient and effective healing, through improvements in healthiness. Health cures injuries better than any medicines.

Cure Tooth Decay: Heal and Prevent Cavities with Nutrition by Ramiel Nagel and Timothy Gallagher

This book presents the important concepts; that healing comes from health and health comes from within. Author Ramiel Nagel claims we can cure cavities – a claim I suspect most dentists would simply not believe. There appears to be no interest in clinical studies to test the assertion. Nagel emphasizes that healing cavities requires improvements in health, not just of the teeth, not just of the mouth, but of the entire body. Unfortunately, because Ramiel Nagel is selling health, not medicine, the material is widely ignored by our corporate bureaucratic product-driven conventional medical establishment.

Effortless Healing: 9 Simple Ways to Sidestep Illness, Shed Excess Weight, and Help Your Body Fix Itself by Dr. Joseph Mercola

This book aims to cure body, mind, and spirit, by improving healthiness. Like most authors, Mercola avoids the stigma of the word cure, speaking instead of healing or using phrases like *side-stepping illness*. The techniques recommended in this book can cure many illnesses. Although the book suggests that results come from aiding healing, many come from improving healthiness. But healthiness is not a medical concept.

The book and Dr. Mercola himself is often dismissed by a medical establishment that has no testable definition for cured and no tools or techniques to evaluate claims of curing.

Transformation

Transformations cure attribute illnesses. Conventional medicine is barely aware of the concept of transformation as a cure. There is little, if any, study into the general concept of transformational cures – even when they are used to produce cures. Many alternative medical practitioners use the word transformation – and most refer to transformation the patient, not some attribute of body, mind, spirit, or community. I find it surprising that surgery, including dental surgery is seldom referred to as a transformational cure, even though it's often referred to as a cure.

Attribute illnesses, except those cured by surgery, are often ignored by conventional medical practitioners, or treated with symptomicines. Surgeries are a cure, but the word cure is seldom used, and tests for cured by surgery appear not to exist. Cures are often expected to be perfect. Transformations are rarely perfect. The concept of negative attributes is poorly studied, even as many illnesses are cured with transformations ranging from minor to incredibly complex cases.

Hospital rehabilitation centers are familiar with many transformational techniques but avoid using the word cure. Cured implies perfection, seldom obtained in rehabilitation. Less severe physical attribute illnesses are often diagnosed, treated, and cured by osteopaths, chiropractors and other alternative practitioners – sometimes by massage therapists, without using the word cure. Priests and psychologists cure many mental and spirit attribute illnesses. Sometimes they are cured by good friends, even by good enemies, who might cure with a whack on the side of the head, physically, mentally, spiritually or communally.

The Pain Cure RX, by Dr. Mitchell Yass: Diagnosing and Resolving Chronic Pain

Describes how to diagnose and resolve many cases of chronic pain, without using the word cure. It is acceptable to tell people how to resolve chronic pain, but not to tell them how to cure chronic pain. Pain, after all, is a symptom, not a disease.

Is the book about cures? Actually, yes. The book is about curing negative attributes of muscles, tendons, and connective tissues, these negative attributes have causes in the past and exist as causes in the present, creating chronic illness. Dr. Yass advises that many illnesses attributed to incurable structural problems like herniated disc are actually due to other issues like muscle weakness or imbalance.

Dr. Yass cures many patients that have been judged incurable or were treated with surgery by conventional medical practice. But conventional medicine does not recognize cures, even as the consequences of their errors are cured. Dr. Yass and his successes are simply ignored by conventional medical systems.

The Body Has Its Reasons, by Therese Bertherat and Carol Bernstein

I bought this book in a used bookstore in Cancun many years ago and found it a joy to read. I occasionally go back for another look. A book about transformation. A book about negative physical, mental, and spirit attributes; blockages, and leakages. A book about how they are created and transformed, although the term used in the book is released. I suspect few people will use it to cure their illness. It is directed at an audience of practitioners, of healers, not to patients. It is a book of anecdotal cures – real cures. A book to stir thinking about cures. It is not written to cure any specific cases of illness.

Pain Free by Peter Egoscue

Peter Egoscue has published several books with the same theme and similar titles, including Pain Free at your PC, and Pain Free for Women.

They can be challenging to read front to back if you are trying to understand a simple problem or to get a general understanding. However, this book is recommended by many physical therapists for chronic pain patients. Therapists often advise patients to study just the section relating to their specific problem and to read and do those exercises. Peter does not claim to cure any pain. But the book presents many techniques which can cure by transforming negative physical or environmental attributes, or by addressing other causes.

Somatics by Thomas Hanna

Somatics is, to my reading, a better presentation, and perhaps an extension of many concepts presented in Peter Egoscue's Pain Free books. Thomas Hanna provides teaching in the concepts of Somatics, so that others can learn from his knowledge and experience. This is a field of medicine and a cure book that should be on every doctor's shelf, in every doctor's head. But it requires touching and manipulating the patient, something many doctors avoid.

I am certain that Somatic techniques can cure many illnesses, but even the simplest cure confuses conventional medical systems. It doesn't cure with medicines or surgery so conventional medicine ignores it completely.

Pain Cure, Pain Free, Somatics, The Body Has its Reasons

The books The Pain Cure, Pain Free, and Somatics present similar concepts and cures for many physical blockages and many conditions currently perceived as disabilities. The Body Has Its Reasons is similar but also attends to negative attributes of mind and spirit.

In each case, the author did their own work, and it appears there is little cooperation or coordination between practitioners of these types of cures. There are no clinical studies of cures, especially with regards to transformational cures. As a result, all three books not are not evaluated by conventional medicine, they are simply ignored. These authors have no peers that are recognized by conventional medical authorities to provide any scientific or medical judgement of their results. As noted earlier, the US/FDA guidelines clearly state that only a drug can claim to cure.

When these practitioners or their techniques produce a cure – nobody cares, except the patient. Patient's claims are not considered reliable. Medical claims are anecdotes, to be ignored.

Too much of today's conventional and alternative medicine operates in commercial silos, and the result is that even when cures occur, they remain hidden from public view and from conventional medical practitioners as well.

Paradox and Healing: Medicine, Mythology and Transformation by Dr. Micheal Greenwood and Dr. Peter Nunn

Paradox and Healing is about transformations or breakthroughs in chronic illness. It is an interesting book looking at illness and cures (although the word cure is not used) in refreshingly innovative ways. However, the authors acknowledge what I noticed throughout the book, with *"As authors, we face a writer's paradox. By writing, especially using traditional vocabulary and syntax, which themselves reflect on our society's value system and logical bias, we are necessarily caught in a trap..."* To define cure scientifically, we need to step away from current medical practice, away from the current concepts of disease, and away from the current medical vocabulary.

The title and the book mix transformation with healing although there is little in the book about healing. Most, possibly all, references to the word healing are references to transformation. Healing can be a cause of or a cure for an attribute illness. Healing is also necessary after many transformations, to complete the cure. This book takes a unique and interesting perspective on health, illness, medicine, and cures.

The Cure for Alcoholism: The Medically Proven way to Eliminate Alcohol Addiction by Roy Eskapa, PhD.

A very interesting book. One that has created a bit of a cure controversy. Author Roy Eskapa claims to provide a cure for alcoholism with the Sinclair Method. Lots of other medical professionals claim it is not a true *"cure"* – without bothering to define cure. There is no doubt that the Sinclair method has cured many patients of alcoholism, but there is also no proof because cured is not defined. Most criticisms I have seen ignore the Sinclair Method and dispute the drug as a cure.

Each side is arguing without a clear definition of cure or cured. Until the terms are defined, there can be no agreement. The cure, the Sinclair Method is a conscious transformation. The patient must take the drug Naltrexone before they begin drinking. The drug stops the downward cycle of addiction that is triggered by drinking alcohol. It prevents the individual occurrences that together create a chronic illness. However, the patient must always have the drug available, and always take the drug before the first drink. They must transform their drinking routine. Once this transformation is in place, the addition fades away. If the transformation fades, or the patient forgets to take the drug, they will suffer a case of alcohol illness – but it is not chronic, not an addiction unless the condition persists. The critics confuse a case of illness with an addiction, a chronic illness. Ray Eskapa claims this cure can be used as a model for curing many other addictions. Maybe he's right. But there is little interest in curing addictions in the conventional medical system. Addictions are treated, not cured. Cured is not defined.

Books that Cure Summary

There are many more books that provide evidence and techniques to cure. However, our ability to judge these books is very weak without a clear definition of cure and cured.

There are thousands of books with cure in the title. Few aim to cure any illness or disease. The word cure is used as a marketing tool. Like click-baiting. Medical books (usually called *"health"* books) often *cure-baiting.* Cured, after all, is not defined. There is no need for scientific rigor. Many books with cure in the title market treatments, with no intention to cure. There are also many books recommending cures, but not using the word cure in their title or contents. They might as well spell cures as ©u®e$™ - copyrighted, registered, trademarked for financial purposes.

Because cure is not defined medically, anyone can claim cure in a book title, and never define the concept, never use the word cure in the contents. Nobody cares. Claims of cure are ignored as meaningless. Today, the word cure has no scientific or medical meaning for most diseases.

Once we develop a clear understanding of the concept of cure as it relates to each type of element of illness, causal illnesses, injury illnesses, and attribute illnesses – we will see these books in a new light. Once we adopt a vocabulary of cure, many will need to be rewritten.

Every true cure works by improving healthiness. Of course, in many cases, we must trade one healthiness for another. Many, perhaps most current medicines work by decreasing specific aspects of healthiness, usually with no attempt to cure. Cures acknowledge and address the causes of illness. Symptomicines, treatments that do not cure, deny the cause, deny the symptoms, deny the illness, and ultimately, deny cures.

With a clear understanding of cure, cures, curing and cured, we can evaluate books that claim to cure, as well as books that claim to reverse disease, prevent disease, roll back disease, help you live with your disease, to more effectively determine which cure and which do not.

Appendix: Definitions

> *How many a dispute could have been deflated into a single paragraph if the disputants had dared to define their terms? --- Aristotle*

The definitions used in this text are healthicine definitions, not medical definitions.

Attribute Illness: An illness caused by the presence or absence of an attribute of diet, body, mind, spirit, or community. An illness with a non-active, present cause. E.g. blocked artery, aneurysm, cataracts, and hernia.

Body: the physical components and attributes of an individual, including the brain.

Calculus: a particular method or system of calculation or reasoning. (Oxford Dictionary).

Calculus of curing: the mapping of a disease, medical condition, or illness to a set of illness elements which can be cured, and those elements which we do not expect to cure, which might be diseases, disabilities, handicaps, signs or symptoms, or perhaps natural features. Only an illness element can be cured, one cure at a time.

Causal Chain: Every cause has a cause, and consequences which might also become a cause, resulting in a chain of causes. Breaking a present causal chain by successfully addressing any individual cause in the chain leads to a cure. Every link in a present causal chain presents multiple opportunities for curing. Analysis of causal chains in the past is useful for preventatives, but usually not useful to cure.

Causal Illness: an illness with a present cause that is part of a life process. E.g. Scurvy, type 2 diabetes, hypertension.

Community: the communities, groups, societies of cooperation that each individual participates in or is a part of – willingly or unwillingly, consciously and unconsciously.

Complex Illness: a group of illness elements with a single cause or causal chain. E.g. A severe Vitamin C deficiency is diagnosed separately as scurvy which can also cause injuries. Complex illnesses are cured by curing each illness element. The sequence of curing can be important.

Compound Illness: a group of illnesses with multiple causes and similar or overlapping signs and symptoms. Many cases of disease are compound illnesses and thus require multiple cures.

Cure: an action that resolves an illness element, or a set of illness elements. Every cure is an individual case, a story, an anecdote.

Cure Element: a cure for a specific element of illness, having a single cause or causal chain, which might be only a partial cure of a complex illness, compound illness, or disease.

Cured: The past tense of cure. The patient cured their own illness.

Cured: The state of having been cured. An illness is cured when the cause and consequences have been successfully addressed such that no more medicines are required for its signs and symptoms.

Curing: working to achieve the end of an illness, one illness element at a time. Curing is often accomplished naturally, by the health of the patient. Sometimes curing requires the assistance of and cooperation with a doctor or other members of the community.

Curable Illness: a negative health condition, which can be cured. An illness is a specific case. Every curable illness consists of a negative judgment that it exists as an illness and a positive judgement that it can be cured. This book is about curable illnesses.

Disease: that which can be diagnosed or that has been diagnosed by a medical professional. Also called a medical condition or disorder. Some illnesses are not diagnosable, therefore not diseases. The concept of diseases is historical and complex, political, not scientific. Some elements of a disease might be curable, while others are incurable.

Healing: A natural cure process that cures injuries to body, mind, spirit, or community and illnesses like the common cold, influenza, and measles which can only be cured by natural process.

Healthicine: the arts and sciences of health and healthiness.

Health: A measurable status of general or overall healthiness.

Healthiness: An individual unit of health. Each unit of health is a whole, consisting of a specific healthiness and corresponding unhealthiness. A measure of healthiness is a measure of wholeness. Every curable illness is a consequence of an absence of healthiness. See: Unhealthiness.

Illness: An illness consists of a cause and its negative consequences. An illness is a hole in a healthiness. An illness is a truth, what the patient has, what the life entity is experiencing that needs to be cured. In this text, the phrase illness generally refers to a curable illness.

Illness Cause: that which, when addressed, results in a cure. Attribution of an illness cause is a judgement tested and validated by curing.

Injury, Injury Illness: an illness with a cause in the past. E.g. A broken arm.

Illness Element: a simple illness, defined by having a single cause or causal chain. An illness element is resolved by an elementary cure.

Mind: the mental functions and attributes, including mental processes, memory, calculation, planning, exploring, understanding and creating.

Placebo and Placebo Effect:
There are many conflicting definitions of placebo and placebo effect in research and literature. In Healthicine, we stick to simple, clear definitions

of each, and clarify with the understanding that clinical placebos are fake placebos.

> *Placebo: a usually pharmacologically inert preparation prescribed more for the mental relief of the patient than for its actual effect on a disorder - Webster's Dictionary*

Placebo: a treatment prescribed by a medical professional with intention to make the patient feel better in some way, but with the belief that the treatment will not cure the patient's illness, will not even improve their condition by itself. Placebos are defined by the intent of the person prescribing the medicine – not by their actual contents or function. A placebo does not exist without the action and specific intent of a medical professional to improve the present health of the patient in some way. Placebos are not necessarily inert.

> *Placebo Effect: improvement in the condition of a patient that occurs **in response to treatment** but **cannot be considered due to the specific treatment used***
> *–Webster's Dictionary*

Placebo Effect: An improvement in the condition or signs and symptoms of the patient following a treatment, where the medical professional does not believe the treatment caused the improvement. Any treatment followed by improvement might be considered a placebo effect by a medical professional who does not understand the cause. Every effect has a cause. When we understand or claim to understand the cause, it is no longer a placebo effect, it is a real effect, with a real cause. A placebo effect cannot exist without the specific opinion of a medical professional.

Clinical Placebo: A fake placebo treatment used in clinical studies. A clinical placebo is fake because:

- the placebo treatment is administered, not prescribed,
- there is no intention to improve the condition of the patient – nor to cure,

- the intent of using a clinical placebo is to test a medical treatment or a placebo treatment, not to address any present cause or illness,
- if the clinical placebo improves the condition of the patient, or cures the patient, the clinical study has failed.

Like a real placebo, a clinical placebo is defined by the persons designing the study, not by its actual contents or properties.

Spirits: the intentions, motivations, passions, goals, attitudes, emotions, and other driving forces of an individual, including spirits of competition and cooperation. Note: this text separates "spirit" from the concept of spirituality, which is linked to religion, not to intention.

Symptomicine: a treatment to address signs and symptoms of an illness with no intention to cure. Most current medicines and medical treatments are symptomicines. Symptomicines can be useful while the health of the patient works to produce a cure, and for incurable diseases, but they can discourage curative actions for illnesses which can be cured.

Transformation: the curing of an attribute illness element by transformation of a negative attribute in diet, body, mind, spirit, community, or environment.

Unhealthiness: absence of a specific healthiness. Health is whole. An individual healthiness and corresponding unhealthiness sum to 100%.

www.ingramcontent.com/pod-product-compliance
Lightning Source LLC
Chambersburg PA
CBHW052142220526
45471CB00004B/1482